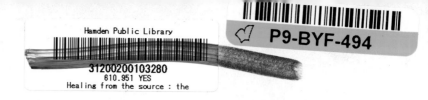
Healing from the Source

Healing from the Source

The Science and Lore of Tibetan Medicine

Dr. Yeshi Dhonden

Translated and edited by
B. Alan Wallace

Snow Lion
Boulder

Snow Lion
An imprint of Shambhala Publications, Inc.
4720 Walnut Street
Boulder, Colorado 80301
www.shambhala.com

9 8 7 6 5 4

Printed in the United States of America

㊿ This edition is printed on acid-free paper that meets the
American National Standards Institute Z39.48 Standard.
♻ Shambhala Publications makes every effort to print on recycled paper.
For more information please visit www.shambhala.com.
Distributed in the United States by Penguin Random House LLC
and in Canada by Random House of Canada Ltd

Library of Congress Cataloging-in-Publication Data
Yeshi Dhonden, 1929–
Healing from the source: the science and lore of Tibetan medicine / Yeshi Dhonden; translated and edited by B. Alan Wallace.
p. cm.
Includes bibliographical references (p.) and index.
ISBN 978-1-55939-148-1
1. Medicine, Tibetan. I. Wallace, B. Alan. II. Title.
R603.T5 Y467 2000
610'.951'5–dc21
99-050958

Contents

Author's Acknowledgments

I would first like to thank His Holiness the Fourteenth Dalai Lama. It is through his dedication to bring a greater awareness of the culture and tradition of Tibet to the world that Tibetan Buddhism and Tibetan Medicine now flourish.

I would also like to thank my teacher, Venerable Dr. Khyenrab Norbu (1883-1962), personal physician to His Holiness the Thirteenth and Fourteenth Dalai Lama (in Tibet), who founded and developed the Men-Tsee-Khang, the Tibetan Medical and Astrology Institute in Tibet.

Special thanks to all those who helped with this book: Alan Wallace for his great skill and commitment to make these ancient teachings available to the modern West, and to those who transcribed and helped edit these lectures, including Dr. Tenzin Dhakpa, Dr. Marsha Woolf, and others.

I would like to thank my staff in India at our clinic: Dr. Lobsang Tenzin, who has been with me for thirty-five years and has acted as my personal attendant, chief pharmacist and director of the clinic. He has not only been invaluable in his service in India, but has accompanied me to America for many years. Together we conducted research at the University of Virginia in 1980, and we are now currently conducting a formal, FDA-approved clinical trial at University of California, San Francisco.

Other staff members to whom I would like to express my thanks include: Venerable Lundup Yeshi, Chomphel Kalsang, Lobsang Tsundu, and Ms. Kalsang Dolma, who serves as my interpreter in both India and the U.S. in our clinical trials.

Finally, I would like to express my gratitude to Dr. Marsha Woolf, who for a number of years has acted as my coordinator in the U.S., liaison and collaborator in the development of our clinical trials, and clinical director.

Dr. Yeshi Dhonden

Translator's Preface

Dr. Yeshi Dhonden was born in Lhasa, the capital city of Tibet, in 1929. His schooling began at the age of six, and two years later he took the novice vows of a Buddhist monk. He began his preliminary studies of Tibetan medicine when he was nine, and at the age of thirteen he was formally admitted to the Astro-Medical Institute in Lhasa. There he studied for five years under the master physician Khyenrab Norbu. His internship lasted from the age of eighteen to twenty-two. For the next ten years, he practiced medicine as an itinerant doctor, traveling widely throughout Tibet. Then in 1959, the year of the Tibetan uprising against the Chinese Communist invasion of their homeland, Dr. Dhonden fled to India, along with 100,000 other Tibetan refugees. In 1961, he became the personal physician of His Holiness the Dalai Lama, a post which he filled for eighteen years. In the following year he re-established the Men-Tsee-Khang, Tibetan Medical and Astrological Institute in Dharamsala, India, where he remained until 1969, when he returned to private practice. The author of *Health Through Balance,* the foremost introduction to Tibetan medicine in English, Dr. Dhonden is among the most renowned of Tibetan physicians living today.

In the editing of these lectures, many people volunteered their time and expertise. I would like to thank all those friends in the San Francisco Bay Area who transcribed Dr. Dhonden's lectures, especially Lynn Quirolo for her unflagging, selfless service. I am also indebted to Dr. Marsha Woolf, David Molk, Loran Davidson, and Kara V. Frame for their help in preparing this manuscript; and I wish to express my special thanks to

Dr. Tenzin Dhakpa of the Tibetan Medical Institute in Dharamsala, India, for his careful reading of the entire manuscript and his many invaluable corrections and comments. Finally, I would like to thank the Balm Foundation for their generous support for the editing of this work.

Introduction

A Brief History of Tibetan Medicine

According to tradition, the fundamental treatises on Tibetan medicine are traced back to the Buddha Śākyamuni himself, making it an ancient discipline, not a recent invention. Buddhism was first introduced into Tibet during the reign of the Tibetan King Thothori Nyentsen, the twenty-eighth king of Tibet (b. 367 CE?), when a casket containing the *Karaṇḍavyūha-sūtra*, devoted to Avalokiteśvara, and a golden *stūpa* fell from the sky onto the roof of Yumbu Lagang, the first royal palace in Tibet.[1] What we now call Tibetan medicine was first introduced into Tibet during the reign of that same king, when two doctors, Biji Gadjé and his female companion Bihla Gadzey, came to Tibet from India and practiced in the court of King Thothori Nyentsen. In Bodhgaya, Tārā, the feminine embodiment of enlightened compassion, had previously appeared to them in a vision and told them they should go to Tibet to practice and teach medicine there. For many generations thereafter, this medical system was transmitted from teacher to disciple solely as an oral lineage, without any textual basis.

King Thothori Nyentsen gave one of his daughters, Yikyi Rölcha, as a wife to Biji Gadjé, who practiced medicine in Tibet for twenty-four years. From their union a son was born named Dunggi Thorchok, so called for

---

1. Tibetans trace their own history as a distinct country with their own royal lineage back 2,123 years. Unless otherwise indicated, footnotes are taken from Dr. Dhonden's lectures.

the white color of his hair, which swirled in a bun on the top of his head. The next seven generations of sons of that line all had the first name of Lodrö, all of them serving as royal physicians. The seventh was Lodrö Shenyen, who served as the personal physician of the father of King Songtsen Gampo (617-650 CE), and his son Khyungpo became the personal physician of Songtsen Gampo himself. This medical system was first put into writing in Tibet during the reign of this king. Khyungpo's son Drejey Vajra traveled three times to India to receive medical training, as did his son Yuthok Yönten Gönpo, who lived to the age of 125 years and served as the personal physician to King Trisong Detsen (742-797). It was during his reign that this medical system first began to flourish widely in Tibet.[2]

King Trisong Detsen was the most important of all the Tibetan kings in terms of bringing Buddhism from India to Tibet in the late eighth century, and it was during his reign that the first Buddhist monastery of Samye was founded. During this era, a great number of Sanskrit manuscripts were translated into Tibetan at Samye. These works set forth the whole of the Buddhist tradition, from the basic teachings of Buddhist monastic discipline, many of the discourses of the Buddha recorded in the *sūtras*, numerous *tantras* revealing the esoteric teachings of the Vajrayāna, and many other fields of knowledge from classical Indian Buddhist culture. This marked the first great flourishing of Buddhism in Tibet.

Moslems from Turkey invaded India in the eleventh century, burnt books on Buddhism and its medical tradition and destroyed Buddhist monasteries. Much of the Buddhist medical literature that had been translated into Tibetan was lost forever in the original Sanskrit. With the recent resurgence of interest in Indian Buddhist literature, Indian and Tibetan scholars in universities in Vārāṇasī and elsewhere in India have been working together to try to reconstruct Sanskrit versions of Indian texts from the precise Tibetan translations.

As for the origins of these teachings, Buddha Śākyamuni attained enlightenment at the age of thirty-five in Bodhgaya in northern India. In his first discourse to five close disciples he taught the Four Noble Truths, setting forth the framework of his entire teachings. Over the

---

2. The royal lineage runs from Songtsen Gampo to Mangsong Mangtsen to Me Agtsom to Trisong Detsen.

following years he gave many discourses, ranging from the basic teachings on ethical discipline to the most esoteric teachings of the Vajrayāna. There are many references to medicine among the *sūtras* and *tantras* that he taught.

Countless eons ago, the Buddha Vaidyarāja appeared on earth and gave many teachings, and he was the first to teach *The Four Tantras.* Buddha Śākyamuni preserved these teachings from the Buddha Vaidyarāja, and he taught them himself in Vārāṇasī. In his text *Vibhāṣākośa* the Indian Buddhist *paṇḍit* Vasubandhu refers to the eight branches of medicine taught in *The Four Medical Tantras* taught by Buddha Śākyamuni when he assumed the form of the Buddha Vaidyarāja in the emanated realm of Sudarśana. In this visionary environment the Buddha, as Vaidyarāja, emanated the form of Vairocana from the crown of his head, symbolizing the primordial wisdom of the absolute nature of reality. From his throat he emanated the Buddha Amitābha, symbolizing the primordial wisdom of discernment. From his heart he emanated the Buddha Akṣobhya, symbolizing mirrorlike primordial wisdom. From his navel he emanated Ratnasambhava, symbolizing the primordial wisdom of equality. And from his genital region he emanated Amoghasiddhi, symbolizing the primordial wisdom of accomplishment.

Rays of light then emanated from his tongue, purifying the verbal defilements of all sentient beings, and upon retracting these light rays, he emanated the personification of the speech of the Buddha, namely Ṛṣi Manasija, who is of the nature of Amitābha and the primordial wisdom of discernment. He circumambulated the Buddha Vaidyarāja three times and requested *The Four Tantras* from him.

Why did an emanation of the Buddha request these teachings from the Buddha himself? At that time the Buddha was surrounded by an entourage of four kinds of disciples: *devas,*[3] *ṛsis,*[4] Buddhists, and non-Buddhists, but they did not have the courage to request of the Buddha these medical teachings. So the Ṛṣi Manasija requested these medical *tantras* from the Buddha Vaidyarāja.

---

3. Translator's note: Tib. *lha.* A "god" within the cycle of existence, who experiences great joy, extrasensory perception, and paranormal abilities, but who suffers greatly when faced with death.

4. Translator's note: Tib. *drang srong.* An accomplished contemplative.

In response, the Buddha Vaidyarāja emanated Akṣobhya from his heart, and he taught the first of *The Four Tantras,* called *The Root Tantra.* Then he emanated Vairocana from the crown of the head, and he taught *The Explanatory Tantra,* the second of *The Four Tantras.* Third, he emanated Ratnasambhava from the navel, and he taught *The Oral Instruction Tantra.* Finally, he emanated Amoghasiddhi from his genital region, and he taught *The Final Tantra.* Although the Buddha Vaidyarāja's speech was but one speech, it was heard differently by each of the four types of disciples. So the *devas* had their own lineage according to what they heard; the *ṛṣis* had their own lineage, and so did the Buddhists and non-Buddhists.

Questions and Responses

QUESTION: Tibetan medicine originated in India, so it must be closely affiliated with, or even have the same origins as, Indian Āyurvedic medicine. If so, what is the relationship now between these two medical traditions?

RESPONSE: These two traditions do indeed have the same origins. When the Buddha revealed *The Four Tantras,* the teachings received and interpreted by the *ṛṣis* grew into the system of Āyurveda. Of course, there was a well-established tradition of medicine in India before the Buddha appeared, just as there was in Tibet before this tradition was introduced there. Both cultures trace their medical history back to very ancient times, but both drew great inspiration from the teachings of the Buddha. However, during first the Moslem and then the British domination of India, much of the Āyurvedic knowledge, literature, and living traditions were lost. In contrast, the Tibetans assimilated these Indian Buddhist medical teachings before the Turkic invasion of India, and—until the Chinese Communist invasion and occupation of Tibet—Tibetan medicine was never suppressed by anyone. The present Āyurvedic and Tibetan medical traditions have much in common, such as ingredients used in medicines, but there are also many significant differences between the two.

QUESTION: It is my understanding that the written Tibetan language was developed as a way to translate the teachings of the Buddha, including both the spiritual teachings and the medical teachings. If that is correct, is it a fairly straightforward process to translate Sanskrit literature into Tibetan, and can original Sanskrit texts that were lost be reconstructed from the Tibetan translations?

RESPONSE: First of all, your initial premise is quite correct. In the seventh century, King Songtsen Gampo sent a number of men from his court, including the most famous Thönmi Sambhoṭa, to India with the order to create a written Tibetan language for the purpose of translating Buddhist literature from Sanskrit into Tibetan. Thönmi Sambhoṭa formulated a Tibetan alphabet and grammar based upon Sanskrit. This made it a fairly straightforward process to translate from Sanskrit into Tibetan. Over the course of time, many translations have been made from Prakrit and Sanskrit into various languages including Chinese, Tibetan, and so on. Generally speaking, from an academic perspective, the Tibetan translations are closer to the Indian original texts than are the Chinese translations, for the Chinese language is radically dissimilar and unrelated to classical Indian languages. The similarity between classical Tibetan and Sanskrit also makes it feasible to reconstruct Sanskrit texts from the Tibetan translations. However, it should be noted that Sanskrit grammar is far more complex than the Tibetan, which does present problems when trying to reconstruct Sanskrit texts from the Tibetan. But on the whole, Tibetan translations from Sanskrit are highly accurate.

As a point of interest, when I was a young boy, around nine or ten years old, an old monk who was my teacher showed me an ancient Tibetan alphabet that he said existed before Thönmi Sambhoṭa created the alphabet we have today. I had never seen anything like this old alphabet, which was unlike either Sanskrit or Chinese. Its boxlike letters were somewhat similar to cuneiform letters in certain Near Eastern languages that I have seen much later in life.

QUESTION: What is the historical relationship, if any, between Tibetan medicine and Chinese medicine?

RESPONSE: That is a very big question, of course. In short, Chinese medicine and Tibetan medicine are radically different in terms of their origins, theories and practices. This is not at all like the relation between Ayurvedic and Tibetan medicine.

However, for many centuries, Chinese emperors invited great *lamas* and physicians from Tibet to their courts, in accordance with the priest-patron relationship that was maintained between the Chinese imperial court and generations upon generations of Tibetan masters. In this way, much Tibetan knowledge was assimilated by the Chinese, which undoubtedly influenced Chinese medicine to some degree. With the recent

Chinese Communist invasion of Tibet, Tibetan medicine is one aspect of Tibetan culture that the Chinese have respected and helped preserve. So now the Chinese are once again making Tibetan medicines according to Tibetan formulas and then selling them in China and abroad as Chinese medicines.

Anyone who reads Tibetan can confirm that the vast majority of the thousands of volumes of Tibetan medical literature are based upon earlier Sanskrit texts, and Tibetan medical treatises commonly pay homage to the Buddha as the source of this tradition. Among Tibetan translations of medical texts, I have seen just one small treatise of fifteen or sixteen verses translated from the Chinese, while all the rest are translated from Sanskrit.

Part I:
The Body in a State of Balance

Chapter One
The Constituents of the Body in Good Health

The Root Tantra is the primary, or fundamental, *tantra*, and it is also the most concise of the four.[5] It consists of six chapters, beginning with a description of the environment of Sudarśana in which these *tantras* were revealed. It then gives an overview of the entire field of Tibetan medicine. The six chapters of this *tantra* correspond to the central metaphor for the whole of Tibetan medicine, namely the tree of medicine, with its three roots, nine trunks, forty-seven branches, 224 leaves, two flowers, and three fruits, each corresponding to specific topics within this medical system. The topics corresponding to the two flowers and three fruits are the professional and spiritual qualities achieved by a totally proficient physician in this tradition.

The first of the three roots, representing the nature of the body, has two trunks, the first of which represents the body that is in good health, when it is said to be in its "unaltered," or natural, state. That trunk has three branches, on which grow twenty-five leaves. The twenty-five topics represented by those leaves explain the differentiation process that takes place during the different phases of digestion, and understanding those topics is crucial for fathoming this medical system as a whole.

---

5. Translator's note: The four primary treatises of Tibetan medicine are called *tantras*, which are the primary scriptures of Vajrayāna Buddhism. A "root" text is a primary, or fundamental, treatise, which generally requires a commentary in order to be properly understood.

The Root Tantra is difficult to understand, for it is very complex and quite cryptic, because it includes so much information in each of its short chapters. Thus, it reads like a collection of lists, with virtually no explication. In these lectures I shall first discuss the body in its unaltered, or healthy state, which corresponds to the twenty-five leaves of the first trunk. I shall include in this explanation all the crucial information about these twenty-five topics by drawing on all four of the medical *tantras*. Once I have given a general presentation of these constituents of the body in good health, I will discuss the nature and origins of illness (symbolized by the second trunk), including the role of the mind and specific mental processes that contribute to disease. In particular, I shall explain the three mental poisons—namely attachment, hatred and delusion—and their role in upsetting the equilibrium of the body and the three humors, which leads to a wide variety of illnesses. The way Tibetan medicine is being taught is improving nowadays due to Tibet's contact with the modern world. In the old days, medical students had to do a lot of rote memorization, without knowing what they were memorizing, but now the traditional texts are being revised so that students are introduced to the meaning sooner.[6]

A general presentation of these twenty-five topics explains many bodily processes, such as retracting and extending the limbs, opening and shutting of the eyes and so forth. When one understands how the various humors, namely wind, bile, and phlegm, function when the body is healthy, one can then comprehend how the humors contribute to disease. Then one is in a position to explore the primary causes and the contributing factors for various types of illnesses.

The twenty-five topics represented by the twenty-five leaves on the first trunk of the first root of the tree of medicine include:

A. Seven Bodily Constituents
　　1. nutriment
　　2. blood
　　3. flesh

---

6. Translator's note: One modern textbook on which Dr. Dhonden draws for this lecture series is the three volumes of the *Bod kyi gso rig slob deb*, by Blo bzang bstan 'dzin (Dharamsala: Bod gzhung sman rtsis khang gso rig mtho slob sde tshan).

      4. fat

      5. bone

      6. bone marrow

      7. regenerative substances

B. Three Waste Products

      1. excrement

      2. urine

      3. sweat

C. Five Winds

      1. life-sustaining wind

      2. ascending wind

      3. pervading wind

      4. fire-accompanying wind

      5. descending wind

D. Five Biles

      1. digestive bile

      2. color-transforming bile

      3. accomplishing bile

      4. sight-giving bile

      5. complexion-clearing bile

E. Five Phlegms

      1. supportive phlegm

      2. decomposing phlegm

      3. experiencing phlegm

      4. satisfying phlegm

      5. connective phlegm

The origins and the natures of the three humors of wind, bile, and phlegm are not discussed elaborately in *The Root Tantra,* but it may be useful to introduce these now for the sake of clarity. The bodies of all creatures on this planet born from a womb are composed of the five elements: earth (solidity), water (fluidity), fire (heat), air (motility), and space. Other life forms, too, such as flowers, consist of these elements. The earth element is the basis from which flowers arise. The water element provides the moisture and fluidity in plants. The fire element is that which provides warmth and leads to maturation of flowers. The wind element produces the growth of any organism, whether it be a flower or a being born from a womb. And finally the space element provides the dimension in which growth can take place. If there were no space, there would be nothing to grow into. Those are the functions of these five elements.

Phlegm has the potency of the earth and the water elements, bile has the potency of the fire element, and wind gives rise to the motion of the blood and the breath within the body. The space element is in evidence in the various cavities within the body, such as the nostrils, the ears, and so forth. These five elements will be discussed in greater detail later on.

If you were receiving the formal, traditional training in Tibetan medicine, you would first memorize long lists of subjects set forth in *The Root Tantra*, before receiving any explanation of them. Only thereafter, when you received instruction on *The Oral Instruction Tantra* and the other two *tantras* would the meanings of those terms and subjects be taught. But I shall explain some of the basic terms and concepts right now.

The locations of the five winds are presented in the following chart:

Winds	Location
life-sustaining wind	crown of the head
ascending wind	chest
pervading wind	heart
fire-accompanying wind	large intestine
descending wind	perineal region

According to the medical *tantras*, the life-sustaining wind is located at the crown of the head, and the pervading wind is at the heart; but according to many other *tantras* within Vajrayāna Buddhism, such as the *Guhyasamaja-tantra*, the pervading wind resides at the crown of the head, and the life-sustaining wind is at the heart. So the positions of those two are reversed.

As a point of interest, the function of the pervading wind is to govern all bodily movements, of extending and retracting the limbs, walking, and so forth. As it is located on the top of the head, it roughly corresponds to the brain, which Western medicine has found to control the movements of the body. According to Vajrayāna Buddhism as a whole, the life-sustaining wind is located at the heart. Moreover, when Tibetans refer to disorders of the life-sustaining wind, we always refer to the heart, which is where such disorders are felt, with symptoms such as heaviness, palpitation, throbbing, and so forth. Thus, even though the medical *tantras* say it is located on the top of the head, in actual practice Tibetan doctors identify it as being located in the heart. So there is somewhat of an incongruity between theory and practice here.

Why then does the Tibetan medical tradition not conform with the rest of the *tantras* in locating the pervading wind in the head and the life-sustaining wind in the heart? The reason is that all Tibetan medical literature is unanimous in its insistence upon the opposite locations for these two winds. Tibetan medical literature consists of *kama*, which are canonical teachings of Buddha Śākyamuni, and *terma*, which are teachings concealed by such masters as Padmasambhava and eventually revealed at the appropriate times. In the course of time, five lineages of Tibetan medicine developed, tracing back to the great Tibetan translator Vairocana, Padmasambhava, Yuthok Yönten Gönpo, Rinchen Zangpo, and Tertön Drapa Ngönshey, who revealed *termas* of *The Four Tantras*. Throughout their development, they did not have much contact with each other. Since all the writings of all these lineages state that the pervading wind is located in the heart and the life-sustaining wind is on top of the head, no Tibetan has had the audacity to contradict them!

I would now like to discuss the twofold category of the components of the body that are subject to being harmed, namely the bodily constituents,[7] and the afflictive elements of the body, namely the humors. There is a mutual dependence between these two. If there were no elements of the body to be afflicted, there could be no afflictions, and if there were no afflictive elements, nothing would be afflicted. These are called the *characteristics of the body*. There are ten afflicted elements of the body, including the following seven bodily constituents and the three waste products:

1. nutriment
2. blood
3. flesh
4. fat
5. bone
6. bone marrow

---

7. The etymology of this term in Tibetan (*lus zungs*) is "body sustainer," for the bodily constituents are the basis for sustaining the body as a whole.

7. regenerative substances (sperm and uterine blood, or ovum)[8]
8. excrement
9. urine
10. sweat

The afflictive elements of the body are the three humors:

1. wind
2. bile
3. phlegm

The interdependence of these ten characteristics of the body and the three afflictive elements are the basis for the formation, sustenance, and eventual demise of the body at death. I shall now address the body when it is in a state of good health. As long as the body is healthy, which is said to be its "unaltered" state, these three afflictive elements, or humors, are supportive of the body, and they perform the various necessary functions for its sustenance and vitality. On the other hand, when the body is in an "altered" state of ill health, these three humors take on the role of afflictions in that they give rise to various types of illnesses, and finally they lead to the dissolution of the body, to death.

The twenty-five components of the body corresponding to the twenty-five metaphorical leaves are first presented within the context of the body in its healthy state, without relating them to the nature and the origins of illness. The ten characteristics of the body that may become afflicted are subject to a fourfold process: (1) digestive warmth, (2) the transformation of food and drink during the digestive process, (3) the results of digestion, and (4) the culmination of the digestive process. The seven bodily constituents are also separated into the two classifications of nutriments and residues. Further subdivisions are made in terms of, for example, the nutriment (or finer portion) and the residue (or coarser portion) of each of the seven bodily constituents, such as the blood and flesh. The nutriment and residue of each of the subsequent constituents are gradually separated following the initial digestive process. Digestive warmth is the primary basis for the transformations of food and drink during the digestive process.

---

8. The Tibetan term (*khrag*) literally means "blood," referring to the uterine blood, but Dr. Dhonden modernizes this term as "ovum" in accordance with modern medicine.

Let us briefly examine the functions of each of the seven bodily constituents and the three waste products. Blood is produced from the nutriment of the food and drink that one ingests. Blood has the function of supplying moisture to the body, it is of primary importance for sustaining the life-force, and it allows for the growth of flesh, which fills out the body. Fat lubricates the body, and the function of the bone is to supply a firmness and structure to the body. The function of the bone marrow is to provide the vital essences for the body, which are closely linked to the body's vitality. The regenerative substances (the sperm and the ovum) have two functions: they give the body its luster, and they are instrumental for procreation.

As for the three waste products, excrement has the function of retaining the subsequent residues in the intestines so that partially digested food is not expelled prematurely, and then it expels the stool. Urine has a similar twofold function with respect to fluid waste products. And finally sweat has the two functions of providing pliancy to the skin and of supporting the growth and maintenance of hair.

The order of the seven bodily constituents relates directly to the progression of the digestive process. When you first ingest food and drink, it takes six days for them to be completely digested and for all of the seven bodily constituents to be produced. The nutriment and the blood are already being produced from the very first day of digestion. Flesh is produced from the nutriment of the blood, and fat is formed in dependence upon the flesh; bone forms in dependence upon the fat; bone marrow is produced in dependence upon the bone; and finally the regenerative substances form in dependence upon the bone marrow. From the time that one ingests food and drink, it takes six days for the regenerative substances to be produced.

Generally speaking, one does not experience immediate effects from Tibetan medicine, and the reason for that is that the medicine has to be assimilated through this whole digestive process. Thus, one will commonly not see the effects of Tibetan medicine until six days after one begins taking it. In contrast, when one takes a modern pharmaceutical drug, this tends to have very swift effects, indicating that it is not being assimilated by way of this entire digestive process. Moreover, when one ingests natural or artificial poisons, they can harm one within an hour or less; for they, too, do not pass through this full digestive process.

To review the functions of the ten characteristics of the body, the nutriment has the function of producing blood, and the blood has the function of nourishing all the moist constituents of the body; and it is the principal support for one's life-force. The flesh throughout the body—on the exterior, the interior, and in-between—may be likened to the plaster on a building. The fat lubricates all parts of the body. The bones function like the pillars that uphold the walls and the roof of a building. The major function of the bone marrow is to supply the body with vital essences. According to Tibetan medicine, the regenerative substances pervade the entire body, so they only roughly correspond to the sperm and the ovum. These substances bring luster to the body, and they are also crucial to the formation of the fetus in the womb. Excrement is located in the large intestine and the rectum, and it has the function of blocking the intestines to support the subsequent residues of the food, which transforms into excrement, and is then evacuated. The major repository for fluid residues is the kidneys. Just as excrement has the function of retaining partially digested food, the urine has a similar function of retaining some of the fluid residues until they have been fully processed. Sweat, once again, has the function of lending pliancy to the skin and supporting the growth of hair. It also has the function of preventing the pores from becoming blocked, which is very important for one's health.

Chapter Two

The Digestive Process

All the transformations of the digestive process are primarily based upon the digestive warmth, which is primarily responsible for the warmth throughout all of the body. To understand what is meant by digestive warmth, we must know its defining characteristics and its role in the digestive process. The digestive warmth that is the basis for digestion is identical to the digestive bile, the first of the five kinds of bile. Digestive bile is crucial for good health and for all the humors and bodily constituents. When the body is in good health, this means that the three humors are in balance. At that time, the function of the digestive warmth is to nourish the body, to prevent disease, and to act as a support for exerting effort. It is the digestive warmth that enhances one's vitality, produces the splendor[9] of the body, and strengthens the bodily constituents.

I would now like to give a brief explanation of the role of the wind humor in the digestive process, and I will later return to this topic in greater detail. From the moment that one puts food into the mouth, the wind humor has a role in digestion, for it retains the food in the stomach so that it does not pass directly into the small intestine. Once the food is partially digested in the stomach by the decomposing phlegm, it moves down to the small intestine, where the gradual segregation of the nutriment from the food begins with the action of the digestive bile, and the

---

9. The "splendor" of the body is especially apparent in people such as professional athletes and others who display a special kind of physical radiance, presence, or majesty.

wind passes the residue down into the large intestine. First, the wind humor has the function of retaining the food in the stomach, like preventing someone from crossing a border until he has the appropriate visa. Once the partially digested food "has a visa" to pass into the small intestine, the wind moves it down to the small intestine, and from there, eventually, into the large intestine.

The function of the digestive bile is literally to "ripen" the food so that it passes properly through the digestive process. When the digestive bile is not functioning adequately, the unripened, or insufficiently processed, food passes directly into the large intestine, which may result in diarrhea. When the digestive bile is functioning properly, it processes the food so that all the bodily constituents are nourished and the body is strengthened. If there were no digestive bile, or if it were not performing its function, then the nutriment would simply not be produced.

In order to digest one's food properly—which means that the digestive bile can properly fulfill its function—one must take good care of this bile by following a healthy diet. For example, one should eat light food that is easily digestible. Heavy food, or food that is hard to digest, will impair the functioning of the digestive bile, which will then hinder the production of the nutriment. In addition, one should follow healthy behavior, for that supports the digestive bile, and this pertains to one's own individual metabolism. There are different types of behavior that are appropriate for people who are dominant in wind, bile, and phlegm. Therefore, it is important to identify the nature of one's own constitution in terms of the three humors, and then learn what types of behavior are especially conducive for one's health. Such wholesome behavior also varies from one season to another. If one conscientiously attends to one's diet and behavior in the appropriate ways, this will enhance the digestive process, which in turn will enhance the production of nutriment, and this will enable one to live a long and healthy life.

Throughout the digestive process, successive segregations are made between the different stages of the nutriment and the residue, each of which is passed on to specific places in the body. In the segregation of the food in the small intestine, the liquid residue turns into urine and the solid residue eventually turns into excrement and moves into the large intestine. Assuming that one's digestion is healthy, until the food is properly digested in the small intestine, the aperture between the small intestine and the large intestine is closed so the food cannot pass on through. While the residue passes into the large intestine, the nutriment from the small intestine goes to the liver. However, if the digestive bile is not functioning properly, the unprocessed food goes into the large intestine. Thus, various types of digestive disorders, including acidity, are due to the improper functioning of the digestive bile. The formation of stomach ulcers due to acidity is caused by inadequate functioning of the digestive bile, such that it does not sufficiently process the nutriment and move it to the liver. As I mentioned earlier, diarrhea may immediately result if the digestive bile is weak, but diarrhea may also result from a malfunction of the descending wind. If the digestive bile and the descending wind are both malfunctioning, this results in flatulence.

The life-sustaining wind moves the food and drink from the mouth down into the stomach. The fluid content of the food and drink one ingests helps disintegrate solid food, and the ingested oils and fats soften the stomach contents. There are three regions in the alimentary canal, corresponding to three phases of the digestive process. The decomposing phlegm is located in the stomach, the digestive bile is located in the small intestine, and the fire-accompanying wind is located in the large intestine. The last is so called because it accompanies the "fire" of the digestive warmth. Like using bellows to increase the heat in a wood-burning stove, the fire-accompanying wind has the function of strengthening the digestive bile. Thus, the digestive bile acts like a fire that "cooks" the stomach contents.

Food and drink have six kinds of tastes: bitter, salty, hot, sweet, sour, and astringent. The life-sustaining wind passes food and drink from the mouth to the stomach, where the decomposing phlegm begins to break them down and homogenize them. At that time, the stomach contents take on a sweet taste and have a bubbly consistency. During this phase, all five types of phlegm are increased and strengthened, which implies that the elements of earth and water in the body, which are closely associated with phlegm, are also strengthened. In the second phase of digestion, in the small intestine, when the digestive bile is doing its work, the contents take on sharp and hot qualities, as well as a sour taste. This phase of the digestive process increases all the five types of bile. In the third phase of digestion, in the large intestine, the fire-accompanying wind has the function of separating the nutriment and the residue. This phase increases the power of all the five types of wind.

My approach in this discussion is to explain the digestive process repeatedly, each time with greater clarity and greater detail. The digestive process first produces nutriment from the food and drink that are ingested, and when the nutriment is well-produced, this is very helpful for the prevention of illness and for longevity. As I mentioned earlier, food and drink are moved from the mouth to the stomach by the life-sustaining wind, and in the stomach it is broken down by the decomposing phlegm, which is of the nature of the two elements of earth and water, and bears a sweet taste. As the stomach contents are broken down by this phlegm, they take on a bubbly quality and a sweet taste. Through this process, the potency of the decomposing phlegm increases (together with the potency of the earth and water elements in the body), which in turn increases the other four types of phlegm as well.

The second phase of digestion takes place in the small intestine, where the digestive bile, which is of the nature of fire, processes the ingested food and drink. Bile is of the nature of the elements of fire and wind, and it imparts to the ingested food and drink a hot and sharp quality and a sour taste (which can be confirmed by removing the contents of the small intestine when they are in this stage of digestion). The digestive bile has the effect of "cooking" the food, and as a result of this process the potency of the digestive bile (together with that of the fire element in the body), as well as all of the other types of bile, is increased.

Once the food and drink have been digested in the intermediate phase of digestion, the fire-accompanying wind separates the nutriment and the digested food. The air element has lightness and motility as its defining characteristics, and it is associated with a bitter taste, so ingested food and drink take on a bitter taste. In this process, the potency of the fire-accompanying wind (together with the potency of the air element in the body), and of the other four types of wind, is increased.

The increase in the humors and elements in the above phases of digestion occurs when the body is healthy, but there is a different description of digestion when the body is ailing. Even after the fire-accompanying wind has done its work, the digestive process is not finished. The above is an account of only the phases of the digestive process in the alimentary canal. There is a lot more to come.

I shall now explain the qualities of digestion. Just as our bodies are composed of the five elements, so is all the food and drink that we take in from our external environment composed of the five elements, and the dominant elements in each type of food and drink determine their tastes. That is, each of the six tastes is determined by the predominance of the individual elements. As we ingest food and drink in which certain elements predominate, yielding their respective tastes, the potency of the corresponding elements within our bodies is increased. This is how the body is nourished. The outer elements from our environment that we take in through food and drink nourish and sustain the inner elements within our bodies.

The earth element that we ingest by way of food and drink increases the flesh and bone, as well as the potency of the sense of smell, enabling one to detect more subtle scents and aromas. The water element ingested by way of food and drink increases the blood and all other fluids within the body, as well as the sense of taste. In this way there is a relationship between the five elements and the six tastes. On the one hand, the earth element always has a supportive quality; the water element has the qualities of fluidity and cohesion; the fire element has the quality of warmth, and the air element has the qualities of lightness and motility. The elements of earth and water both pertain to phlegm, which is associated with a sweet taste. Generally speaking, a sweet taste is present because of the predominance of the earth and water elements. This is discussed in much greater detail in *The Explanatory Tantra*.

The fire element, which pertains particularly to the digestive bile, has the general function of imparting warmth to the seven bodily constituents. Wherever there is warmth in the body, this is due to the fire element. In particular, this element enhances the blood, which is to say, it nourishes the liver, for the liver produces the blood. In addition, the fire element enhances the visual faculty: it enables one to see more clearly. Foods such as black pepper, bell pepper, and chili are all dominant in the fire element.

The element of air[10] is especially associated with a bitter taste, and ingesting food and drink in which this element predominates enhances the sense of touch. The air element is generally responsible for all type of

---

10. Translator's note: There is just one Tibetan term for "air" and for "wind," namely *rlung*.

movement and growth in the body, including the circulation of the blood, the movement of all other bodily constituents, the growth of hair, and so on. Finally, the element of space pervades all of the preceding elements of earth, water, fire, and air. It allows for all types of cavities and openings within the body, including the pores, and it enhances the sense of hearing.

Questions and Responses

QUESTION: What is the relation between the digestive bile as it is described in this system and bile as it is understood in modern Western medicine?

TRANSLATOR'S RESPONSE: Translating such material is a multi-phased task. The translator's first responsibility is to give a literal and accurate rendering in English of Tibetan medical terms. For example, the first of the five types of bile is called in Tibetan *mkhris pa 'ju byed.*[11] The first part of this term, *mkhris pa,* is commonly translated as *bile.* The final two syllables *'ju byed* mean *that which digests,* or simply *digestive.* So the translation of *digestive bile* is a straightforward, literal translation from the Tibetan, without reference to Western medicine. Similar, literal translations are given for the other subclassifications of the humors.

Once the literal meanings of individual terms are properly understood, we can begin to understand them within the context of Tibetan medicine, which in many respects is radically different from Western medicine. That is the second phase of translation: to comprehend the meanings of specific terms within their own theoretical framework.

As for the third phase, once one has understood the meaning and significance of digestive bile, for instance, according to Tibetan medicine, one can begin to explore how this relates to other theories concerning the digestion, such as Western medicine's own understanding of bile as a secretion of the liver. But it is not feasible to proceed to this third phase of understanding unless one has already completed the first two phases. My chief task here is to make advances primarily in the first two phases, then later researchers can build on such work to develop the third level of comparative understanding.

---

11. Translator's note: Pronounced "tripa jujé."

Very often, when translating technical medical terms from the Tibetan tradition, the translations, such as *wind, bile,* and *phlegm,* are likely to be misleading, especially for those who are well versed in the meanings of these terms according to other medical systems. Thus, when first encountering these translations, it is best to take them simply as temporarily empty ciphers, without relating them to one's prior associations with these words. To ensure that students of Indian and Tibetan medicine do just that, some translators refuse to translate the three humors into English and instead leave them in Sanskrit as *vāta, pitta,* and *kapha.* This certainly has the advantage of dissociating them from one's previous associations and preconceptions, but it also indicates a refusal to rise to the task of translation.

QUESTION: What is your justification for translating the three humors as *wind, bile,* and *phlegm?*

TRANSLATOR'S RESPONSE: The reason for translating these terms in this way is that ancient Greek medicine (which influenced Tibetan medicine by way of Persia), early Roman medicine, and subsequently medieval European medicine all have humoral theories that lend themselves to comparison with the Tibetan humoral theory. The Āyurvedic medical tradition of India, with which Tibetan medicine is most closely affiliated, also incorporates a theory of the three *doṣas* of *vāta, pitta,* and *kapha,* which are commonly translated as *wind, bile,* and *phlegm.* Moreover, there is certainly some relation between the Tibetan concept of phlegm and bile and the modern medical meanings of these terms. But there are enormous differences as well. While bile, for example, is regarded in the West as a fluid secreted by the liver and stored in the gall bladder, according to Tibetan medicine, bile has a much more diverse range of meanings.

QUESTION: I suspect that the Tibetan medical definition of good health may be different from good health as it is conceived of in Western medicine. According to Tibetan medicine, doesn't good health imply not only physical health but also a happy, balanced, stable mind? How do you understand the differences between Tibetan and modern Western notions of good health?

RESPONSE: I will respond briefly to this question now, but this will be addressed directly or indirectly as I continue in this presentation of Tibetan medicine. Generally speaking, Tibetan and modern Western notions of good health correspond fairly closely. The nature of good health, or the body in its unaltered state, is discussed in three chapters of *The Explanatory Tantra.* Maintaining good health depends in large part on one's behavior. In this regard, one difference between Tibetan and modern scientific medicine is that the latter tends to give general health tips concerning diet, exercise, and so on that all people are encouraged to follow. In the Tibetan tradition, in contrast, advice for maintaining good health is more specific, relating to an individual's specific humoral constitution. Someone may be, for example, a wind-dominant person, or a wind-bile-dominant person, a phlegm-dominant person, a phlegm-bile-dominant person, and so on. First, people are encouraged to identify the nature of their own individual constitution, and then they are taught to follow advice specific to their bodies, which may be inappropriate for many other people.

QUESTION: In the West a person who is strongly influenced by the mental affliction of attachment or anger may be regarded as quite healthy, but from a Buddhist perspective, such a person is unwell. Isn't this an important difference between these two perspectives on good health?

RESPONSE: That's quite true. Tibetan Buddhism has a lot to say about mental health and spiritual maturation. But this is true not only of Buddhism and Tibetan culture. Rather, all over the world there are people who recognize that the normal mind is not very healthy. Many people in the West today—some of them adhering to no religion, some Christian, and some of other faiths—acknowledge that the mind afflicted by attachment, anger, and delusion is not well. Isn't this an insight shared among many people throughout the world? Many people, too, have discovered that one can improve the normal mind to make it healthier. So Buddhism does not stand alone on these issues. I will return to this topic later on.

QUESTION: From what you have explained of Tibetan medicine so far, I see that it is a complex and sophisticated system, but in the West how can one tell who is really qualified to practice Tibetan medicine?

RESPONSE: From one perspective, this is indeed difficult. In Tibet qualified physicians had earned a degree, or certificate, from one of the two major Tibetan medical colleges, indicating that they had successfully undergone the entire training in this discipline, passed the final examinations, and were now qualified to practice. This is similar to the modern Western tradition of earning degrees and licenses indicating one's competence in a certain field. In the modern West, which has had little contact with Tibetan medicine, it's very difficult to evaluate those who claim expertise in this field, even among those who do have some kind of certificate of training.

In Tibet there were three levels of degrees that one could earn as a result of one's medical training. The highest is the Rapjampa degree, the middling is the Bumrampa degree, and lowest is the Kachupa degree. All those who earn any of these degrees must, at the very least, have memorized all *The Four Tantras* verbatim. In addition, one who receives the highest degree must be thoroughly familiar with the *Blue Vaiḍūrya,* a commentary to these *tantras* composed by the Regent Sangye Gyatso in the seventeenth century, as well as many other treatises from all the lineages of Tibetan medicine. This means that one has memorized all these texts verbatim and has fathomed their meaning through a lengthy process of logical analysis and debate with other students and doctors. The Bumrampa degree is conferred upon those who have mastered roughly one half the texts required for the Rapjampa degree. The textual knowledge required of one who receives the Kachupa degree is simply the memorization of all *The Four Tantras,* but not many of the commentaries on these texts. Nowadays there are quite a few young Tibetan physicians who have sound textual knowledge, but little practical experience in this discipline. True mastery of Tibetan medicine comes not only from book learning but from years of post-graduate study, treating patients, and working with the herbal compounds used for treating all manner of illnesses.

The Transformations of the Nutriment

The process of separating the nutriment and the residue begins once the partially digested food and drink have been passed down into the small intestine. After the completion of digestion in the small intestine, the residue turns into two aspects: solid and fluid. The solid residue becomes excrement, and the liquid residue becomes urine. Recall that the decomposing phlegm breaks down the stomach contents, the digestive bile digests them, and the fire-accompanying wind separates the nutriment from the completely digested food and drink. The fluid part moves through very small channels from the small intestine to the portal vein and to the blood vessels and then to the kidneys, where it becomes urine. The solid portion of the residue goes from the small intestine to the large intestine, where it moves to the rectum, which is a kind of holding place. It is then expelled from this location when one defecates. The fluid residue makes its way from the small intestine to the kidneys and then on to the urinary bladder, which is like a little pot, where it is stored.

Each of the seven bodily constituents has its own warmth, which is imparted to it by the digestive bile. The first nutriment, which is produced in the initial segregation of the nutriment from the residue, transforms into blood. The nutriment of the blood transforms into flesh; the nutriment of the flesh transforms into fat; the nutriment of the fat transforms into bone; the nutriment of the bone transforms into bone marrow; and the nutriment of the bone marrow transforms into the regenerative substances. Due to the warmth of each of the bodily constituents, the decomposing phlegm, the digestive bile, and the fire-accompanying wind are each activated in each of these subsequent transformations, further separating the nutriment from the residue with respect to each of these seven bodily constituents.

The classic texts on Tibetan medicine state that the nutriment passes from the small intestine to the liver by way of nine channels. To explain what is meant by this, fluid in an unbaked clay pot does not flow out all of a sudden, but rather slowly seeps out the vessel. Likewise, the nutriment seeps through a permeable wall from the small intestine to the liver. Once it gets inside the liver, it does move through distinct channels to the portal vein and then to the blood vessels.

In the liver, the nutriment is transformed solely into blood due to the activation of the same three humors mentioned earlier, namely the decomposing phlegm, the digestive bile, and the fire-accompanying wind. The nutriment of the blood transforms into flesh, and the nutriment from that eventually turns into fat. In each of these phases there is a separation of the nutriment from the residue. As I mentioned, the nutriment of the fat transforms into bone, and the nutriment of the bone transforms primarily into bone marrow, but also into the brain, the spinal cord, and cartilage.[12] The nutriment of the bone marrow goes to the "vesicle of regenerative substances," which refers to the seminal vesicle in

---

12. It also transforms into the senovium, but that is not explicitly mentioned in the classic texts.

men and to the ovaries in women. In Tibetan there is one term for these two parts of the body. In this vesicle the nutriment turns into the regenerative substances, namely the semen and ovum. But the segregation process is not yet finished. There is still one more segregation to take place.

The nutriment of the regenerative substances consists of minute particles, each of which is no larger than a sesame seed. These move from the vesicle of the regenerative substances up to the life-force channel in the heart. This corresponds to a channel in the back of the heart through which blood flows, and which is linked to the other channels going to the lungs and other organs. The nutriment of the regenerative substances is located in the life-force channel. This is the finest, most subtle of the nutriments that are produced throughout this entire digestive process. Within the life-force channel this nutriment is located between two elements: a white element above, and a red element below. These two elements are like two cups enclosing the nutriment between them. This nutriment is the primary support of all the bodily constituents, and it is the most crucial factor for longevity, vitality, health, and for the splendor of the body. The region of the life-force channel in which it is located is about a half inch in length. This channel is behind the heart, not actually in the heart itself. The residue of the regenerative substances turns into the "red element" and the "white element." In men, the white element is equivalent to the semen, which is stored in the seminal vesicle. In women, the red element is the ovum, which is located in the ovaries. Small amounts of the red and white elements from the vesicle of regenerative substances also go up to the heart, where they enclose the most subtle nutriment, the potency of which pervades the entire body, even including the hair.

Questions and Responses

QUESTION: In the case of sudden death due to an accident or a wound in battle, what happens to the nutriment stored in the life-force channel behind the heart?

RESPONSE: According to the Tibetan medical tradition, if one's body is pierced in a vital organ—such as the liver, the heart, or the brain—with a spear, an arrow, or a sword, one will die, for no treatment will prove effective. In that case the nutriment that resides in the life-force channel behind the heart loses its potency immediately, and it can no longer pervade and thereby support the entire body and all the bodily constituents. However, if one is stabbed in the small or large intestine, one may recover with proper treatment. There are recorded cases of this in the medical treatises of ancient India and Tibet. However, if one is deeply wounded in any of the vital organs in the upper abdomen and chest, this will likely prove fatal. Part of the reason for that is that all the processes of separating the nutriment from the residue, as described earlier, can no longer occur, and that results in death.

QUESTION: The cases just described are all ones in which the body has been pierced deeply by things such as a sword and so forth. What about a case of impacting, as in a fall?

RESPONSE: This is basically similar to being pierced by a sword and so on. If the impact is so severe that one can no longer breathe, the effect on this most subtle nutriment is the same; and the whole process of separating the nutriment from the residue can no longer occur. In such circumstances, death occurs so abruptly that it is not really possible to apply one's meditative abilities to the dying process. However, in cases in which one dies gradually, there are techniques with which one can meditate on the specific phases of the dying process, attending to the successive visions that occur in this process. One is taught to anticipate these different phases so that one can become fully cognizant of each one, and enter with full consciousness into the transitional process following death. In this way, it is possible to transmute the entire dying process into a meditation, which has a great benefit after this life.[13]

In the case of death due to a violent impact or piercing, one does not have this opportunity, for death is too abrupt. In such a case, either immediately or up to four days after the fatal trauma, one's consciousness will depart from the body and enter into the *bardo,* or intermediate state, following death, in which one's experiences take on a dreamlike quality. During that period, one has a mental body, as one does in a dream. But there are differences between this intermediate state and the dream state: while in this intermediate state, one can witness the physical

13. Translator's note: Such practices are described in detail in Sogyal Rinpoche's *The Tibetan Book of Living and Dying* (San Francisco: HarperSanFrancisco, 1992), Part Two.

world experienced by living beings. For example, one can hear conversations taking place in this physical world, but most living people cannot detect the presence of such a being in the intermediate state. Moreover, at least at the beginning of this period, one is not aware that one has died. One feels that one is still alive and that people should see and hear one, but they don't and this is very upsetting.[14]

QUESTION: In the case of a gradual death as a result of internal causes, is there a comparable experience in this *bardo,* or intermediate state?

RESPONSE: Yes, it is the same. You can see and hear events in the physical world, but the living do not see or hear you.

QUESTION: In the case of a gradual death resulting from internal causes, once you are in the intermediate state, are you unaware that you have died?

RESPONSE: This is a complex issue, for there are many differences from one person to the next. If one is a Buddhist practitioner, there are a lot of things that can be done if one has the good fortune to experience a gradual death. First of all, one looks for the proximate signs indicating that one will die soon. In this way one already begins to anticipate one's dying process. When the dying process actually begins, a well-trained person will already have learned how the various elements in the body lose their potency, one by one. Moreover, one may have trained in meditation to anticipate these phases of dying, by rehearsing for them, so to speak. When one begins to die, that which one has rehearsed previously in meditation is applied to one's present experience. Now one anticipates and recognizes each of the phases of the dying process as the elements lose their potency, one by one. One has already learned the different types of visions that arise—the white vision, the red vision, and the black-out—so one is fully cognizant of the entire dying process.

With the withdrawal of the potency of all the physical elements, a pale white vision, a reddish vision, and penultimately a blackout occur. After the blackout comes an experience called *the clear light of death.* If

---

14. Translator's note: For a detailed description of the intermediate state see *Death, Intermediate State and Rebirth in Tibetan Buddhism,* Lati Rinbochay & Jeffrey Hopkins (Ithaca: Snow Lion, 1985).

one has sufficiently trained in meditation, when this clear light of death manifests, one may recognize it for what it is. If so, one may attain spiritual awakening, or enlightenment, in the aspect of the *dharmakāya*.[15] In that case, one does not enter the intermediate state. Most people experience the clear light of death without recognizing it, and they proceed into the intermediate state. They still have the opportunity to recognize the intermediate state for what it is, and if they do so, they may achieve enlightenment in that state. Such people are said to attain enlightenment in the aspect of the *sambhogakāya*.[16]

Moreover, for people who are well-trained, when entering the dying process it is possible to direct, or transfer, one's consciousness from this life to a destination of one's choice. Tibetan Buddhists generally transfer their consciousness to a *buddha*-field, where they dwell in the presence of a *buddha*, receive spiritual teachings, and progress towards enlightenment. If one has trained in the *illusory body*, the realization from such practice can also be applied to the dying process. Following the death of one who is adept in such practice, the body actually shrinks down to two feet in length, or even smaller. This has actually occurred in Tibet during the last ten or fifteen years. Even since Tibet has been under Chinese occupation, some Tibetans secreted themselves in caves up in the mountains, and while the Chinese were destroying Tibetan culture, they continued to practice meditation in solitude. Over the past decade or so, some of those who have accomplished this have died in Chinese prisons, witnessed by their fellow inmates. I have seen a book recently written by a Tibetan who saw this and called the Chinese guards to witness it for themselves. The guards reportedly came and examined the shrunken body of such an adept and saw for themselves that it had not been artificially altered in any way. This is a recent event witnessed not only by Tibetan Buddhists, but by Chinese who have no religious beliefs at all.

Over the last 1200 years in Tibet, many people are reported to have gone beyond even that stage of practice, and at their death their gross

---

15. Translator's note: Cf. *Natural Liberation: Padmasambhava's Teachings on the Six Bardos*, comm. by Gyatrul Rinpoche, trans. by B. Alan Wallace (Boston: Wisdom Publications, 1998), Ch. 6.

16. Translator's note: The *sambhogakāya* is a subtle, archetypal form of an enlightened being, which is apparent only to other *buddhas* and highly realized beings known as *āryabodhisattvas*. Cf. *Natural Liberation: Padmasambhava's Teachings on the Six Bardos*, Ch. 8.

material bodies simply vanish, leaving only the fingernails and hair behind. They are said to have achieved the rainbow body, but that requires a great deal of practice. There is much more that can be said about this.[17]

The Transformations of the Residue

Having explained the entire sequence of distillations of ever finer nutriment, I shall now discuss the complimentary process of the gradual segregations of the residue. The residue includes the phlegm of the stomach, which goes to the bile and to the cerumen in the ears, eyes, nose and so on. Some of the residue also turns into body oil in the pores, intestinal gas, teeth, sweat, the nails, the oily lining of the intestines, head hair and body hair, and finally the regenerative substances. In the final segregation, the most subtle nutriment goes up to the heart, and the grosser residue remains in the vesicle of regenerative substances, that is, in the seminal vesicle for men and in the ovaries for women.

The residue of food and drink in the small intestine turns into excrement and urine as explained previously, while the nutriment goes to the liver. In the liver a further segregation takes place, the residue of the blood goes to the gall bladder, and the residue of the flesh turns into sebum (which emerges from the pores) and cerumen (which emerges from the eyes and ears). The residue of the fat turns into sweat and body oil. The residue of the bone turns into the teeth, nails and hair on the body and head. The residue of the marrow becomes the oily lining of the intestines that allows the stool to pass. This residue also appears as an oiliness around the nose and ears, and around the rectum, where it facilitates the passage of the stool. In the segregation that occurs in the spine, the nutriment goes to the heart, while the residue turns into the red and white elements, which are equivalent to the ovum and sperm. One ancient view within the Tibetan medical tradition is that sweat is a residue of all of the seven bodily constituents, but other schools differ on this point.

The most refined nutriment, which is located in the life-force channel behind the heart, supports one's vitality and health, enhances the complexion, and it produces the splendor of the body. While it is located in this channel behind the heart, it pervades the entire body, and it is the basis for all experiences of happiness and physical well-being.

---

17. Translator's note: Cf. Sogyal Rinpoche's *The Tibetan Book of Living and Dying*, pp. 167-169.

As I explained previously, from the time that one ingests food and drink, it takes six days to produce the most refined nutriment that goes to the heart. There are exceptions to this rule, however, as in the case of ingesting poisons and aphrodisiacs. In ancient Tibet there was a tradition of making aphrodisiacs that allowed for the production of the regenerative substances in one day. Myrobalan, which is a general antidote to poison, also has an immediate effect. Most herbal medicines begin to produce their therapeutic effects within one day. Most foods generally take six to seven days to be completely processed, but there are some exceptions. Some foods are lighter and easier to digest, while others are heavier and slower to digest. Moreover, if one's body is very weak or emaciated, then milk and meat juice may also produce an immediate effect upon the body.

During that six-to-seven-day process, on the first day blood is produced; on the second day flesh is produced; on the third day fat is produced; on the fourth day bone is produced; on the fifth day bone marrow is produced; and on the sixth day the regenerative substances are produced, with the finer nutriment going up to the heart.

There are various types of naturally occurring poisons, such as the corrosion that forms on certain types of metals such as brass and copper, the full effects of which may take years to manifest. In addition there are artificial, manufactured poisons. In some of the border regions between Tibet and Assam there were tribes who concocted deadly poisons that would result in death only after three years. The effects of such poisons were so subtle that the victims did not know they had been poisoned, but they would gradually lose their vitality and finally pass away.

Most herbal medications for disorders of the three humors begin to have their effects within one day. There is, as it were, a self-sustaining cycle of the seven bodily constituents. The food and drink one ingests turn into the bodily constituents, which allows one to continue eating and drinking.

Chapter Three
The Humors

The Classification of the Humors

This explanation of the classification of the humors of wind, bile, and phlegm includes a discussion of (1) the subclassifications of the humors, (2) their causes, (3) their essential natures, (4) an analogy, and (5) the result of humoral imbalances.

(1) The five kinds of wind are the life-sustaining wind, the ascending wind, the pervading wind, the fire-accompanying wind, and the descending wind. The five kinds of bile are the digestive bile, the color-transforming bile, the accomplishing bile, the sight-giving bile, and the complexion-clearing bile. The five kinds of phlegm are the supportive phlegm, decomposing phlegm, experiencing phlegm, satisfying phlegm, and connective phlegm. These fivefold classifications refer to the principal types of humors, but there are more subtle variations among them. There is a more detailed classification of 404 diseases, but they are all included among disorders of the five winds, five biles, and five phlegms.

(2) The threefold classification of the humors is derived from their primary causes, namely the three mental afflictions of attachment, hatred, and delusion. Attachment is the primary cause of imbalances of the wind, hatred produces imbalances of the bile, and delusion is the primary cause of phlegm imbalances.

(3) The essential nature of these three humors is that they sustain the body when it is in good health; but when it is in ill health, the humors produce heat and cold disorders.

(4) As an analogy, according to Indian Buddhist astronomy, that which obscures the sun and moon during eclipses is an entity called Rāhu. There is a detailed explanation of the nature of eclipses in the great commentary to the *Kālacakra-tantra* called *The Stainless Light.* Rāhu dwells in space even when there is no eclipse, and this is like the effect of the humors on the body when one is in good health. But the obscuration of the sun or moon during an eclipse is like the injurious effect of the humors upon the body when the body is in an unbalanced state.

(5) The result of the humors when they are out of balance is disease, and that is why the literal meaning of the Tibetan term translated as *humor* is *defect* (*nyes pa*).

The remedies for the three humors of wind, bile, and phlegm are the earth element, water element, and the fire element, respectively. For example, if one is suffering from a wind disorder, it is helpful to eat rich, highly nutritious food. For a bile disorder, one should eat cool food, and for phlegm disorders one should eat warming food that has a strong element of heat.

In terms of the periods of the day and night, wind disorders tend to arise at dawn and in the evening; bile disorders tend to manifest at midnight and at noon; and phlegm disorders tend to arise in the morning and at dusk. In terms of the seasons, wind disorders arise in the summer, or rainy season; bile disorders arise in the fall; and phlegm disorders arise in the spring.

In terms of the phases of the digestive process, phlegm disorders are most likely to arise immediately after the ingestion of food or drink; bile disorders tend to arise when the food is being digested; and wind disorders most frequently arise when the digestion is complete.

In terms of the different elements, the nature of wind is the air; the nature of bile is fire; and phlegm is cool and of the nature of earth and water. The wind humor is variable in the sense that if a heat disorder occurs, wind becomes hot; whereas if a cold disorder occurs, it becomes cold. Thus, wind is regarded as being like a trouble-maker who roams about taking on the bad qualities of his associates. The wind is likened to a rogue, for when an imbalance of any of the humors arises, the wind invites it in, and facilitates it from the beginning. Thus, the wind exacerbates all humoral imbalances. In the case of a fatal imbalance of the humors, it is the wind that ends one's life by stopping the breath. So the wind is a culprit in all these cases, like a rogue who looks for mischief wherever possible.

As for the diversity of disorders, there are few kinds of bile disorders, but if one does arise, it tends to have a sharp and swift effect. For example, if one is afflicted by a heat disorder that is dominated by the bile, it can quickly become deadly. There are also relatively few phlegm disorders, and they act slowly. The wind humor acts like bellows to enhance whatever type of disorder arises, exacerbating both heat and cold disorders. A wide array of diseases are caused by organisms, and their variations of heat or cold disorders depend on the bile or phlegm that is affected. These too are exacerbated by the wind humor. Just as wind disorders tend to arise quickly, so do herbal remedies for such disorders work quickly.

Questions and Responses

QUESTION: You said the wind pervades the entire body and exacerbates any illness that arises. If you have a phlegm disorder or a bile disorder, in addition to prescribing a remedy for that, would you also prescribe a medicine for the wind that is exacerbating the imbalance?

RESPONSE: The standard procedure when giving Tibetan medicine is to give three different types of medication per day: in the morning, afternoon, and evening, pertaining to the relative dominance of each of the humors throughout the day. In so doing, wind is taken into account. For example, a bile disorder is an imbalance in its own right; it is not wholly sustained by the wind humor. So if the predominant ailment is a bile disorder, that is the primary focus of the treatment. For a heat disorder, cool and dull[18] medication is prescribed to balance that. But by taking cool and dull medication, one may exacerbate a wind disorder, for coolness corresponds to a quality of wind. All this must be held in balance. To make sure that as a result of that first medication you don't counter the heat disorder and at the same time exacerbate a wind disorder, you would complement the first medication with a second that has an oily quality. The medications prescribed throughout the course of the day should bring balance to all the humors. This is unlike most Western medication, in which a single remedy is prescribed for a specific ailment. Such a single-track approach often leads to unwanted side-effects. By prescribing three medications throughout the day, such side-effects can be avoided from the beginning.

---

18. This quality (*rtul ba*) is both soft and cool.

QUESTION: How can one enhance the "splendor" of the body, and if it diminishes, how can one restore it?

RESPONSE: The splendor of the body diminishes because of disorders of the three humors, so one restores the splendor by balancing the three humors, bringing them back to a state of equilibrium. If the humors are already in equilibrium, there are herbal tonics that one can take to increase one's vitality and thereby enhance the splendor of the body. In Tibet it is very cold, especially in the winter, so some of the tonics prescribed there consist largely of butter. But if these were taken in a warm climate, they would be unhealthy. So a medication that acts as a tonic in one climate may be detrimental in another.

QUESTION: Apart from following a healthy diet, are there other techniques, such as meditation or exercise, to enhance the finest nutriment stored in the life-force channel?

RESPONSE: You should first see that you are following an appropriate diet. To do so, you need to check out your own metabolism and determine which humor or humors are dominant. Then your diet should be adjusted to balance your humors. That will enhance the nutriment at the heart. Moreover, the type of exercise you practice should also be appropriate to your own humoral constitution. Those are the medical ways of enhancing this nutriment.

The stages of life, the consistency of the stool, and the locations of the humors also pertain to this question. Understanding these points will help you live in such a way that this nutriment will be enhanced by your diet and exercise. There are three chapters in *The Explanatory Tantra*[19] that pertain to different types of behavior, namely, routine conduct, seasonal conduct, and incidental conduct. Here you will find a discussion of diet and conduct aimed at increasing vitality in general and specifically the nutriment at the heart.

Meditation is an entirely different realm of practice. If you wish to practice Vajrayāna Buddhism, you must first receive a tantric initiation, which empowers you to engage in various types of meditation. In Tibet solitary recluses would retreat high into the mountains to meditate, with

19. Translator's note: Cf. *The Quintessence Tantras of Tibetan Medicine*, trans. Dr. Barry Clark (Ithaca: Snow Lion, 1995), Chs. 13-15 of *The Explanatory Tantra.*

no access to food, so they would live on "vital essence" pills, which are high-nutrition, herbal compounds that are empowered by meditation. If one succeeds in this practice of empowering such pills, one can live indefinitely on just three of these pills a day, without ingesting any other food at all. If one hasn't achieved a fairly high degree of meditative realization, it is unlikely that one will succeed in this practice, so I generally do not give them to those who request them.

The Formation of the Bodily Constituents in the Womb

The primary cause of the humors of the developing fetus is the three humors from the parents, which are initially conveyed to the developing fetus by way of the regenerative substances. These three humors are of the nature of the four elements. The male and female regenerative substances are of the nature of the five elements (including space), and they have within them the three humors, which are themselves of the nature of the three poisons of attachment, hatred, and delusion. In addition, when the fetus initially forms, the very subtle consciousness of a being from the intermediate state prior to this life enters into the union of the sperm and ovum. This subtle stream of consciousness is conjoined with a very subtle, invisible continuum of the five elements. This subject is very difficult to comprehend in terms of modern science, which has focused on the nature of the physical world, while largely ignoring the nature of consciousness. The consciousness that enters the union of the sperm and ovum cannot be detected by scientific means. The regenerative substances of the parents have in them the three humors, and at conception they are conjoined with this consciousness that comes in with its own habitual propensities from previous lifetimes. Those habitual propensities include imprints of five types of mental afflictions: attachment, hatred, delusion, jealously, and pride. In their ordinary state, these five mental afflictions generally harm the individual, and among them, the three poisons discussed earlier give rise to disorders of the humors. When these five mental afflictions are sublimated and purified, they manifest as the five types of primordial wisdom of an enlightened being.[20]

---

20. Translator's note: These are the primordial wisdom of the absolute nature of reality, mirrorlike primordial wisdom, the primordial wisdom of equality, the primordial wisdom of discernment, and the primordial wisdom of accomplishment.

How is it that the male and female regenerative substances, which are the primary cause of the formation of the fetus, can be imbued with the three humoral imbalances? And while the fetus is forming, how can it develop in conjunction with these humors that are of the nature of the three poisons? This may be understood by an analogy: There are certain types of wood that are deadly poison, but certain insects in that wood feed on it and are not harmed by it. Like such insects, these same three humors that lead to illness when they are out of balance also facilitate the development of the fetus when they are in balance.

The mother's diet and conduct influence the type of metabolism that her baby will have. For example, if she ingests food and drink that are predominately of the nature of wind, and likewise if she engages in conduct that increases the power of the wind humor, this will cause her baby to become wind-dominant. Likewise, if she takes food that increases bile and engages in bilious conduct, this will contribute to her baby being bile-dominant. The same is true for food and behavior pertaining to phlegm.

There are seven types of humoral constitution. People may be dominant in (1) wind, (2) bile, (3) phlegm, (4) wind-bile, (5) wind-phlegm, (6) bile-phlegm, or (7) they may have equal proportions of wind, bile, and phlegm. It is best to have the seventh kind of metabolism. In terms of the size of one's body, a wind metabolism will give rise to a small body, a bile metabolism will give rise to a medium size body, and a phlegm will give rise to a large body. The three twofold combinations of the humors give rise to medium-sized bodies.

As for the degree of warmth in the body, a wind person has unstable warmth, a bile person has strong warmth, and a phlegm person has little warmth. This warmth is closely related to the digestive warmth, which determines one's ability to digest food, and for a developing fetus this is influenced by the diet and conduct of the mother. These are the characteristics of people who are dominant in one or more of the humors. A wind-dominant person finds it difficult to defecate, a bile-dominant person, who is of a hot and sharp nature, has loose, fluid bowels, making it easy to defecate. Compared to a wind- or bile-dominant person, a phlegm-dominant person, being of the nature of the elements of earth and water, finds it moderately easy to defecate. The consistency of the stool also pertains to the three seasons: the hot season, the rainy season, and the cold season. It also pertains to the three stages of life: childhood, adulthood, and old age.

The General Locations and Functions of the Humors

To review the general locations of the three humors, phlegm is located in the upper part of the body and especially the brain; bile is in the mid-portion of the body and particularly the liver and gall bladder; and wind is in the lower region of the body, particularly the hips and waist. When the body is healthy, the wind humor, though located in the hips and waist, moves in all the bones, ears, skin, heart, life vessels, and the large intestine. Those regions also correspond to the passageways through which disorders of the wind pass. In a healthy body, bile moves in the blood, sweat, eyes, liver, gall bladder, and intestines. These regions also correspond to the passageways of bile disorders. Finally, in a healthy body phlegm, though located in the brain, moves in the nutriment, flesh, fat, bone, marrow, regenerative substances, excrement, urine, nose, tongue, lungs, spleen, stomach, kidneys, and urinary bladder.

Pertaining to the healthy body, there is a twofold discussion of the general and specific functions of the humors. The general functions of the wind are inhalation and exhalation, moving the limbs, and expelling and retaining waste products, such as urine, excrement, and mucus. Pervading the whole body, wind also moves all the seven bodily constituents as well as the three waste products. It is generally responsible for participating in all types of mental, verbal, and bodily activities. Another general function of the wind is to bring clarity to all the five senses, and it enables one to identify with one's body, providing one with a basis for one's personal identity.

Bile, which is of the nature of fire, is responsible for hunger and thirst and has the function of ingesting and digesting food. Bile also has the function of producing all the warmth throughout the entire body and giving one a clear complexion. Moreover, just as the sun ripens fruit, so does the bile "ripen" the seven bodily constituents and bring them color. Bile gives one a sense of courage, determination, and fortitude, and it also leads to aggression and resentment, which may be directed towards others or oneself in a self-destructive way. This is due to the connection between bile and hatred. In addition, bile enables one to exert effort and have ambitions, it acts as the basis for the four kinds of intelligence—deep, fast, sharp, and subtle—and it enables one to think ahead.

Phlegm, being of the nature of earth and water, lends strength to all of the constituents of the body, and it give stability to one's intelligence and awareness as well. A bile-dominant person tends to have a sharp memory and great pride, such that if he comes up with an idea and gets right to it, he will accomplish it; but if he delays, he will likely shift to some other idea or plan. In contrast, a phlegm-dominant person is tenacious, and tends to carry through with anything he undertakes. Phlegm acts as the basis for memory, and it has a carefree quality such that one does not become anxious over trivial circumstances. For example, a phlegm-dominant person is likely to remain calm in a crisis. If a phlegm-dominant person is injured by someone once or twice, he is not likely to retaliate, but will probably respond in a jovial way. But if such a person is repeatedly harassed, he will eventually retaliate fiercely. Phlegm has the general function of connecting and lubricating all the joints, and it produces the softness, oiliness, and pliancy of the body. In addition, having a ponderous quality, it has the general function of bringing about mental stability, as well as drowsiness and sleep. A phlegm-dominant person likes to sleep and is uncomplaining and forbearing with respect to hunger and thirst. If deprived of food or drink for a long time, such a person does not whine or complain, but simply forebears until nourishment is obtained. In general, a phlegm-dominant person is able to endure much suffering.

Questions and Responses

QUESTION: My question is about the interaction between the habitual propensities of the incoming consciousness that joins with the sperm and ovum at conception and the humoral constitutions of the parents. If both parents have dominant bile constitutions but the incoming consciousness has strong propensities for attachment, what is the outcome?

RESPONSE: In that case, the fetus will have a combined wind-bile constitution, influenced by wind from its own prior stream of consciousness and by bile from the two parents.

QUESTION: Which of these two influences has a stronger influence on the humoral constitution of the developing fetus?

RESPONSE: If the parents, especially the mother (whose influence is stronger than the father's), are dominant in bile, and the incoming consciousness is dominant in attachment, the fetus will have a bile-wind constitution, indicating a stronger constitutional influence by the parents. Like-

wise, if both parents are dominant in wind and the incoming consciousness has strong propensities for hatred, the fetus will have a wind-bile
constitution. The first humor listed in such a combination (bile-wind
versus wind-bile) indicates that it is primary.

If one is a bile-wind-dominant person, the qualities of sharpness, anger, and irritability supersede the qualities associated with wind. While
the humoral dominance of the regenerative substances themselves su-
persedes the propensities of the incoming consciousness, the influence
of the regenerative substances is superseded by the diet and conduct of
the mother during gestation. That has the strongest influence on the
developing fetus' constitution.

QUESTION: Should a pregnant mother alter her diet and conduct from
what it was prior to the pregnancy?

RESPONSE: Generally speaking, no. However, since a threefold humoral
constitution is optimal, it would certainly be beneficial for a pregnant
mother to adjust her diet and conduct accordingly. In fact, that was frequently done in Tibet: expecting mothers would alter their diet and conduct to balance their own constitutions so that their baby would develop
in the most healthy way. Moreover, during the first eight months of pregnancy, it is important for the proper development of the fetus that the
mother not allow her blood to be taken and that she does not take emetics.

In Tibet, if a couple was incapable of conceiving a child, a doctor
would examine both the man and woman. If the problem was on the
man's side, medication would be given to "purify" the male regenerative
substance. If the problem was on the woman's side, she would be given
fertility medication. In addition, other medication might be taken shortly
after conception to determine the gender of the child. For example, if a
woman wanted a boy, she could take a medication to determine that gender for her infant, and she might also recite *mantras* and follow a prescribed diet and conduct to aid the proper development of the fetus. Much
of this knowledge has been lost in Tibet since the Chinese occupation.

QUESTION: Does the Tibetan tradition have birth control medications?

RESPONSE: Yes. The formulas for these are found in the classic medical
treatises, but these would be given only to people who already had many
children. It was prohibited to give such medication to people who simply

didn't want to have any children. The rationale behind this prohibition was religious: according to Tibetan Buddhism, human life is considered to be extremely precious and to engage in sexual intercourse and yet deprive a sentient being from taking such a rebirth is considered to be selfish. There was never any population problem in Tibet. There were six million people distributed over one million square miles of Tibet before the Chinese invasion.

There are two types of birth control in Tibetan medicine: one to prevent conception permanently and the other to prevent conception only temporarily. I personally do not make the medication that permanently inhibits conception, but I do prepare medications that temporarily block conception, which is primarily aimed at preventing annual pregnancies.

QUESTION: Is any birth control medication given to men?

RESPONSE: No, only to women.

QUESTION: If a person is born with a predominance of one or more of the humors, is it possible to alter that predominance over the course of one's life by regulating one's diet and conduct?

RESPONSE: No, that is not possible. This is why it is said that the diet and conduct of the mother during pregnancy is so important, for it determines the humoral constitution of the child for rest of its life.

QUESTION: Even if the qualities associated with the different constitutional types can't be eliminated over the course of a lifetime by one's diet and conduct, isn't it possible to transform, or sublimate, traits such as anger, hatred, and aggression by spiritual practice, so that they manifest in beneficial, rather than detrimental ways?

RESPONSE: Yes, that is indeed possible.

QUESTION: What general types of diet and conduct facilitate humoral balance?

RESPONSE: One should not eat exclusively hot, salty, or bland foods, but rather eat moderate amounts of a variety of foods. Likewise, in terms of one's daily conduct, one should neither constantly engage in extremely demanding, arduous work or remain lethargic. Seek moderation in your entire diet and behavior.

The Specific Functions and Locations of the Humors

The Five Types of Wind

Having explained the general locations and functions of the three humors, I shall now give a more detailed account of the specific functions and locations of each of the five kinds of wind, bile, and phlegm. Beginning with the five winds, the life-sustaining wind is located on the crown of the head, but it moves from there, through the throat and chest, down as far as the solar plexus. It functions principally in the channels, bones, and the brain, and it contributes to swallowing food and drink, inhaling and exhaling, expelling saliva and mucus, and facilitates the process of sneezing. It also contributes to the clarity of the mind and senses and to attentional stability.

The ascending wind is located in the bones just above the solar plexus. Its functions pertain to the nose, tongue, uvula, and esophagus, for it contributes to verbal articulation. Furthermore, it contributes to the general strength, radiance and complexion of the body, bringing clarity especially to the ruddy and pale hues of the complexion. Finally, it is responsible for all types of exerting effort, and it maintains one's mindfulness and powers of recollection of one's actions and concerns pertaining to the past, present and future.

The pervading wind is located in the heart, but it pervades the entire body including the internal organs, the five sense faculties, and the seven bodily constituents out to the pores of the skin. Once food and drink have passed through the three phases of digestion in the alimentary canal, the pervading wind distributes the nutriment throughout the various bodily constituents. Moreover, it has the function of moving the major and minor limbs, including walking and all other types of movement. It also opens and closes all of the orifices of the body such as the eyes. Generally speaking, all the movements of the body occur in dependence upon the pervading wind.

The fire-accompanying wind is located in the large intestine, as may be recalled from the previous discussion of the three phases of digestion in the alimentary canal; but it also moves through the stomach, the small and large intestines, and throughout all the cavities in the body. Its principal function is to segregate the nutriment from the residue. It also "ripens" the ten afflicted elements of the body—namely, the seven bodily constituents and the three waste products—and generally causes growth throughout the body.

The descending wind is located in the perineal region and extends upwards as far as the lower portion of the thoracolumbar fascia that lines the spinal column. It is also moves in the male and female genitals, the large intestine, the urinary bladder, the seminal vesicle, the ovaries and uterus, and the thighs. Its function is to expel and retain the male and female regenerative substances, the fetus, menstrual blood (the older blood is expelled while new blood is being produced), urine, and excrement. Moreover, if the fetus dies in the womb, the descending wind expels it, and at birth it also expels the placenta.

The Five Types of Bile

The most complicated and important of the five types of bile is the digestive bile, which is located in the small intestine, between the areas where the food is undigested and where it has been digested. In terms of its functions, it digests the food, and it plays some role in differentiating the nutrient from the residue. It produces all the warmth in the body; even the warmth produced by the four other types of bile arises in dependence upon this bile, which supports all the rest. It also contributes somewhat to the transformation of color within the body, and it is responsible for drying up ingested fluids within the body. Finally, it is responsible for producing hunger and thirst.

The color-transforming bile is located in the liver, but it courses through all the bodily constituents, including the nutriment, the blood and so forth. It creates the colors of all of the bodily constituents, especially the red and white colors in the body. For example, it makes blood red, the bones white, and it provides color to the hair. In addition, it produces the warmth in all the internal organs.

The accomplishing bile is located in the heart. It prevents attentional scattering, sustains attentiveness, and supports the stability and clarity of one's intelligence. Ambition, effort, and determination, as well as one's sense of personal identity, arise in dependence upon the accomplishing bile.

The sight-giving bile is located in the eyes, and it enables one to see external forms, including shapes and colors, and spatial dimensions, and it also provides one with the ability of subtle discernment.

The complexion-clearing bile is located in all the pores of the skin. Its function is simply to bring a clarity to the complexion of the skin. If you have a good complexion, that is due to this bile.

The Five Types of Phlegm

The supporting phlegm is located in the chest, specifically in the breast bone and the upper ribs to the left and right of the breast bone, perhaps corresponding to the xyphoid. It supports all the other four types of phlegm, and it performs the functions of all the fluids of the body. Moreover, it supports the elements of earth and water throughout the body.

The decomposing phlegm is located in the stomach, where the food is still undigested. It has the function of decomposing the ingested food and drink, congealing them, and sending them on to the next phase of the digestion, where they are processed by the digestive bile.

The experiencing phlegm is located in the tongue, and it has the function of experiencing all the six types of tastes.

The satisfying phlegm is located principally in the head, but it functions from the base of the neck upwards. It has the function of bringing satisfaction to the five senses as they perceive their various objects.

The connective phlegm is located in all the major and minor joints. It has the function of connecting and lubricating all the joints, which provides them with a pliancy so that one can extend and retract the major and minor limbs.

Among the three humors, wind, being of the nature of the air element, has the characteristics of being rough, light (the opposite of heavy), cold, thin (i.e., it is able to course through very narrow passages), hard, and motile. Bile, being of the nature of the fire element, has the characteristics of being sharp, oily, hot, light, odorous, purgative and moist. Phlegm, being of the nature of the earth and water elements, has the characteristics of being oily, cool, heavy, dull, smooth, stable, and sticky.

The wind humor is imbued with neither strong warmth nor coolness. Nevertheless, when it works in conjunction with bile, it aids the bile in the production of warmth. When it works in conjunction with phlegm, it aids phlegm in producing heaviness and coldness. Pervading all parts of the body, it facilitates both warmth and cold, so it is said to be neutral, though it is a bit cool. Bile is simply hot, and phlegm is cold.

Questions and Responses

QUESTION: Are the characteristics of the three humors principally tactile in nature?

RESPONSE: Yes, that is true.

QUESTION: Does the function of the sight-giving bile pertain to the need of some people to wear glasses?

RESPONSE: Yes, there is a relationship between poor eyesight and the sight-giving bile. If the elements of water and earth become too predominant in the body, they stifle the production of heat, which leads to liver problems. This is a very complex topic, but poor eyesight can often be attributed to inadequate liver functioning, which in turn adversely affects the kidneys. When the liver is malfunctioning, this obstructs the functioning of the color-transforming bile. The fundamental problem here is the inadequate production of warmth in the body due to the digestive bile. As a result, other types of bile, such as the sight-giving bile and the color-transforming bile, are also not able to function properly. As a result, the earth and water elements become predominant, and that gives rise to a predominance of phlegm. Phlegm then accumulates in the kidneys, and this leads to problems of the eyesight. In short, the problem stems from the liver, then passes on to the kidneys. In addition to poor eyesight due to problems in the liver and kidneys, there are thirty-two maladies of the eyes themselves.

QUESTION: The pervading wind and the accomplishing bile are both said to be located in the heart. Are they located in the heart as a whole, or do they reside in specific chambers within the heart?

RESPONSE: The pervading wind and the accomplishing bile both reside in the heart as a whole, not in specific chambers within it. The Tibetan medical *tantras* say that the pervading wind resides in the heart, but according to all the other Buddhist *tantras,* such as the *Vajramālā Tantra,* the pervading wind is located in the crown on the head and not in the heart. In colloquial Tibetan people say that a person's brain is confused or that someone has a really good brain. When referring to a person's intelligence, we generally refer to the brain and not the heart, though we do associate the heart with memory. This way of speaking corresponds to all these other *tantras* that say the pervading wind resides in the head. Despite this difference between the medical *tantras* and other Buddhist *tantras*, they all agree that the pervading wind pervades the entire body.

QUESTION: Are all skin disorders—including skin cancer, skin ulcers and so forth—due to a malfunction of the complexion-clearing bile or to other factors?

RESPONSE: The preceding discussion relates to the body in its unaltered, or balanced state. The complexion-clearing bile is related to various types of skin disorders, but there are many other contributing factors as well. Specifically, if the earth and water elements become too predominant, this obstructs the functioning of the various forms of bile, including the complexion-clearing bile, which not only hampers the complexion but may contribute to more serious skin disorders. When the body is in an imbalanced state, any one of the three humors may be excessive, deficient, or disturbed. As a result of any of these humoral problems, various skin disorders and many other diseases may arise.

QUESTION: In the Chinese medical system, the type of energy called "*qi*" is fundamental not only to the body but to the universe in general. Do any of the constituents of the body you have discussed thus far correspond to this kind of energy?

RESPONSE: The five elements are integral to the physical constitution of your own body, to all other living organisms, and to the universe as a whole. Those elements are closely related to the three humors. Like Chinese medicine, Tibetan medicine also includes the practice of acupuncture and moxibustion. Tibetan medical treatises also discuss various methods of surgery, but in practice they were abandoned centuries ago in Tibet. Briefly stated, the Chinese term *qi* is related to the Tibetan word *loong* (*rlung*), which is our word for the air element and the wind humor. The Tibetan medical tradition originally includes five types of medical treatment, including moxibustion, blood-letting, the application of hot and cold poultices, immersion in hot springs or mineral water, and finally a wide variety of massages with and without the use of oils. From Tibet they were brought to Mongolia and from there to China. The Chinese are now very proud of these techniques and claim them as their own heritage, but they received them indirectly from Tibet.

QUESTION: What is the relationship between "the indestructible *bindu*," often mentioned in Buddhist *tantras*, and the most refined element of the nutriment?

RESPONSE: The "indestructible *bindu*" is identical with the most refined nutriment, which gives rise to longevity, strength, and so forth.

The Humoral Constitutions

Human anatomy is understood first of all in terms of gender, which includes male, female, and hermaphrodites (individuals who have both male and female genitals). Secondly, the human body is classified in terms of age. According to the Tibetan tradition, the first age group is from birth to the age of sixteen, and that is called "childhood." The next age group is from sixteen to seventy, and that is called "adulthood," implying that all one's bodily constituents and sensory faculties are increasing and are strong during this phase of life. The age bracket from seventy upwards is called "old age," and during this phase, one's bodily constituents are no longer increasing. From the age of fifty upwards, one's blood is no longer being produced as it was previously, and the menstrual cycle ceases. But it is generally said that up until the age of seventy, one is still in one's prime.

The nature of the body is classified in terms of the dominant humors and humor combinations. This is determined during gestation by one's mother's diet and conduct, the predominance of specific elements in the fetus' own body, and by the *karma* of the unborn child. This entails a sevenfold classification, namely, a body that is dominant solely in (1) wind, (2) bile, (3) or phlegm, dominant in (4) both wind and bile, (5) phlegm and bile, and (6) phlegm and wind, and (7) a body that is strong in all three of the humors. I shall now give a more detailed account of each of these constitutions of people who are in good health.

(1) Wind has many functions but no form of its own, and a corresponding characteristic of wind-dominant people is that they have a small and slender stature, their posture is slightly stooped, and when they move, their joints tend to make a crackling sound. Their complexion tends to have a bluish tinge, they are sensitive to cold and wind, and they prefer warm and cozy places. They are loquacious, talking about all manner of things, mixing meaningful conversation with pointless comments. They

generally have little wealth or material enjoyments, and they have rather short life spans. They do not sleep very much, they are light sleepers, and are easily aroused from sleep. They are "party people," who love song and dance and enjoy others doing the same. They are easily aroused to laughter, but they also are prone to being quarrelsome. They are gregarious and sociable, for if they are alone they have no one to talk to. In terms of their food preferences, they like sweet, sour, bitter, and hot food.

Wind-dominant people are said to have some characteristics in common with vultures, foxes, and crows in the following ways. Vultures fly to great heights and distances, and they are energetic. Likewise, wind-dominant people tend to be active, energetic, mobile, and light on their feet. They are also like foxes, who are always on the move, sniffing all kinds of scents, and frequently digging up anything that catches their interest. Finally, such people are likened to crows, who will eat almost anything, are aggressive, and have harsh voices.

(2) People who are dominant solely in the bile humor tend to have strong appetites even shortly after eating and drinking. This is because they have much heat in their bodies, while the water element is deficient. Their hot characteristic causes them to be very thirsty, and their sharp quality gives them strong appetites. They also tend to digest food and drink quite quickly, which also accounts for the fact that they are hungry and thirsty soon after eating and drinking. Their hair and complexion tend to be ruddy or yellowish, which is due to the fire element.

I suspect many Westerners are bile-dominant. Such people have sharp intelligence and can act quickly. There is nothing sluggish about them. Their personalities are generally sharp, and they have sharp memories and attention. They tend to be proud, conceited, and egotistical, thinking they are in a class by themselves. Consequently, they resist taking orders from anyone, and they are very capable of looking after their own interests. Because of their dominant fire element, they tend to perspire a great deal and to be malodorous. Fire is unstable, for it is constantly flickering (it is neither as unstable as air nor as stable as water or earth). Thus, bile-dominant people tend to have middling life spans, middling degrees of wealth, and medium statures. In terms of their food preferences, they like sweet, bitter, and astringent tastes, and cooling foods. They are prone to having strong cravings. Bile-dominant people are likened to tigers, monkeys, and *yakṣas,* a type of demon that is very fond of flesh and blood. Such people are like tigers in that they are energetic and aggressive. Like monkeys, they are sharp-witted, quickly responsive, and light on their feet. And, like *yakṣas,* they are proud and conceited.

(3) Phlegm-dominant people have cool bodies with round contours, for their joints are concealed by flesh, and they tend to obesity. Because they are predominant in the water and earth elements, they have fair complexions, free of blemishes, and they are not easily aroused to hunger or thirst. Their posture is erect. Because of the quality of inertia of the earth element, such people are forbearing, so they can maintain emotional equilibrium even when they are harassed, when things go wrong, and when they do not get their own way. They generally have amiable dispositions and are good-natured. If they are aroused to such emotions as craving, anger, or pride, they express them only gradually. They are not impulsive. Because of the predominance of the water element, they are able to endure considerable heat, and due to the predominance of the earth element, they can endure strong hunger and thirst. They tend to have great wealth and large physical frames, they sleep long and deeply, and they have long life spans. They appear to be easygoing, and when they do feel anger or pride, they tend to hold them inside. They may quietly bear grudges for years on end before they finally retaliate, and when they do so, they strike back with a vengeance. As for their food preferences, they like hot, sour, and astringent tastes, and they like coarse food. Phlegm-dominant people are likened to lions, elephants, and lead buffaloes. Like lions, they have great strength and longevity, and they often outshine others. Like an elephant and a lead buffalo, they have great strength.

(4-7) On the basis of the preceding descriptions of wind, bile, and phlegm-dominant people, one can infer the qualities of people who are dominant in wind-bile, bile-phlegm, and phlegm-wind, as well as people who are equally strong in all three humors. Among the three dual dominant humors, wind-bile-dominant people tend to have the smallest physical proportions, wealth, and life span. Phlegm-wind-dominant people generally have a middling stature, wealth, and life span; and bile-phlegm-dominant people are likely to have relatively large physical proportions, wealth, and life spans. Among those seven categories, it is best to be equally dominant in all three humors.

One's humoral constitution is determined during the formation of the fetus, and it remains that way for the rest of one's life. It is determined first of all by one's *karma,* the habitual propensities from the previous actions of the being in the intermediate state who is about to be conceived. The second factor is the relative dominance of any of the three humors of the male and female regenerative substances that are united at conception. Thirdly, during the first seven months of the development of the fetus, the diet and conduct of the father and especially the mother are extremely important influences. For instance, if the mother eats very fatty foods, this will give rise to a predominance of bile in her developing fetus. If she eats a lot of heavy and sweet foods, this will give rise to a predominance of phlegm in the developing fetus. Nevertheless, the principal factors that determine one's humoral constitution are the *karma* and the habitual propensities from previous lifetimes that are brought to this life by the being in the intermediate state who becomes conceived in the mother's womb.

This concludes a general discussion of the twenty-five leaves representing the bodily constituents, waste products, and humors when the body is in an unaltered state.

Part II:
The Body in a State of Imbalance

Chapter Four
An Overview

While the first trunk of the metaphorical tree represents the body in its unaltered, healthy state, the second trunk represents the body when it is in a state of imbalance. On this second trunk the first branch represents the primary causes of disease. The second branch represents the contributing conditions for the arising of illness. The third branch represents the entrances through which the illnesses come into the body. The fourth branch represents the locations of the humors. The fifth branch represents the passages through which the illnesses move. The sixth branch represents the ages, environments, and seasons in which various illnesses arise. The seventh branch represents the results of diseases. The eighth branch represents combinations of humoral imbalances. The ninth and final branch represents a synthesis of all the proceeding. There are further subclassifications, but I will not go into those now.[21]

There are three leaves on the first branch, which represents the primary causes of disorders, namely attachment, hatred, and delusion. Since time immemorial, the fundamental cause of suffering is ignorance, which is the root cause of the three mental poisons of attachment, hatred, and delusion. Attachment is the primary cause of wind disorders; hatred is primary cause of bile disorders; and delusion is the primary cause of phlegm disorders. These three are called *poisons* because they kill our progress along the path to spiritual liberation.

---

21. Translator's note: Charts of all the roots, trunk, branches, and so forth of the tree of medicine are presented in the *Encyclopedia of Tibetan Medicine*, Vaidya Bhagwan Dash (Delhi: Sri Satguru Publications, 1994), Vol. I, pp. 113-136.

The second branch represents the contributing conditions for the arising of disorders, of which there are four types. The first contributing condition is seasonal change, the second is demonic influences, the third is diet, and the fourth is conduct.

As for the third branch, there are six such entrances through which disorders enter the body. Diseases may first penetrate the pores of the skin, expand in the flesh, move through the channels, cling to the bones, and descend upon the five solid organs and the six hollow organs. The five solid organs are the heart, lungs, kidneys, liver, and the spleen. The six hollow organs are the stomach, gall bladder, small intestine, urinary bladder, vesicle of regenerative substances, and the large intestine.

The fourth branch, representing the location of illnesses, concerns the locations of the imbalances of the humors. On the one hand, such disorders occur everywhere throughout the body. However, phlegm disorders predominantly occur in the brain, and they are related to the water and earth elements and to delusion. Bile disorders, which are related to heat, the element of fire and to hatred, occur in the mid-portion of the body, specifically in the liver, the gall bladder, and the diaphragm. Wind disorders, which are associated with the air element and the mental affliction of attachment, occur predominantly in the hips, waist, and large intestine. The three leaves representing the predominant locations of phlegm, bile and wind correspond to the upper, mid, and lower regions of the body.

As for the fifth branch, there are fifteen passageways through which imbalances of the humors move. Wind disorders travel through the bodily constituent of the bones, through the sense faculty of the ears, through the sense field of tactile sensations, through the solid organ of the heart, with its life-force channel, and through the hollow organ of the large intestine. Bile disorders travel through the bodily constituent of the blood, the waste product of the sweat, the sense faculty of the eyes, the solid organ of the liver, and the hollow organs of the gall bladder and small intestine. Phlegm disorders travel through the bodily constituents of the nutriment, flesh, fat, bone marrow, and regenerative substances, the waste products of the excrement and urine, the sense faculties of the nose and tongue, the solid organs of the lungs, spleen, and kidneys, and the hollow organs of the stomach and urinary bladder.

When the body is in an unaltered condition, the twenty-five components of the body—the seven bodily constituents, the three waste products, and the five categories of wind, bile, and phlegm—are not excessive, deficient, or disturbed. Then the body is in good health, and the humors enable the complete digestive process to function properly, such that the nutriment is transformed into blood, and so on. That, in turn, enables one to have a long life. On the other hand, an altered condition of the body occurs when one or more of the humors is excessive, deficient, or disturbed, or if one's diet or conduct is unhealthy. To understand the body in its altered state, one must identify the causes and contributing conditions for illnesses.

I shall discuss the nature of illness in terms of five topics: (1) the causes of illness, (2) the conditions contributing to illness, (3) the manners of entrance of illnesses, (4) the characteristics of humoral imbalances, and (5) classifications of diseases. The fundamental question addressed in this discussion is: what is to be healed? The simple answer to that question is: the imbalances in the body which arise in dependence upon the five aggregates, namely physical form, recognition, feeling (including pleasure, pain, and indifference), compositional factors (including a wide array of mental processes), and consciousness (the five sensory types of consciousnesses as well as mental consciousness). The first of these aggregates is physical, while the latter four are mental in nature.

Due to an excess, deficiency, or disturbance of any of the ten afflicted elements of the body (the seven bodily constituents and the three waste products), the three humors are not able to function properly. Conversely, an excess, deficiency, or disturbance of any of the three humors brings illness to the ten afflicted elements. Moreover, if any one of the three humors is in a state of imbalance—being either excessive, deficient, or disturbed—this results in imbalances in the other humors. For example, an excess of bile suppresses phlegm, which then becomes deficient. There is an interrelationship among the humors and the bodily constituents. Thus, if steps are taken to correct an imbalance of one, this may create a reciprocal imbalance of others.

Chapter Five
The Distant Causes of Illness

There are two types of causes of illness: distant and proximate, and among the distant causes of illness, there are general and specific causes. According to the Buddhist world view, since beginningless time we have had innumerable bodies, not all of which were human. We have taken rebirths as a wide variety of sentient beings, including animals. Throughout the course of these many lifetimes we have repeatedly killed and devoured one another. The full range of the general, distant causes of illness is inexpressible, for these span innumerable eons during which, in our previous lifetimes, we have been subject to the three mental poisons of attachment, hatred, and delusion. Consequently, we have been born as all species of animals, human beings, and many other classes of sentient beings. Therefore, it would be impossible to list every single one of these general, distant causes of illness.

Nevertheless, all these innumerable distant causes of illness stem from one fundamental cause. According to Buddhism, out of ignorance, sentient beings reify their own independent, inherent personal identities, which in reality do not exist; and that ignorance, known as *self-grasping*, is the fundamental, distant cause of illness. To repeat this point, in reality the self does not exist as an independent, inherent entity, but under the influence of ignorance, we compulsively reify ourselves as being inherently existent, and that is the root cause of illness.

As an analogy, wherever a bird flies, it is inevitably accompanied by its own shadow. It can never fly so fast or so far that it escapes its shadow. Similarly, as long as one is subject to this ignorant tendency of reifying oneself, one is vulnerable to illness. The primary cause of illness is present, so all that is needed is for it to be activated by contributing conditions. While everyone wishes for long life, happiness, health, and well-being, as long as one reifies oneself, one will never be free from illness. In brief, as long as one is subject to ignorance, it is impossible to be invulnerable to illness.

The common causes of illness include both outer and inner phenomena. The outer causes are such things as weapons, rocks, accidents, collisions, and so forth. The inner causes are the three humors: wind, bile, and phlegm. In dependence upon those outer and inner causes, an innumerable array of diseases arises in the body.

There are many methods for counteracting self-grasping, but there are obstacles to such practice as well. First, most people would not believe there was any point to them even if they took the trouble to learn them. Most non-Buddhists would not accept their validity, and even many Buddhists, who ostensibly believe in them, give them only lip service, without actually implementing those methods.[22]

Buddha Śākyamuni was previously an ordinary person like ourselves, but through his quest for truth he discovered means for counteracting and eliminating self-grasping and thereby attaining spiritual awakening and liberation from the source of suffering. To understand the methods for counteracting self-grasping, one must become familiar with the Four Noble Truths: the truths of suffering, the source of suffering, the cessation of suffering, and the path to the cessation of suffering. The actual methods to counteract and eventually eliminate self-grasping are included in the truth of the path to the cessation of suffering. These methods, in essence, consist of ethical discipline, meditative concentration, and the cultivation of wisdom. On the basis of leading an ethical life, one stabilizes the mind in meditation, and then cultivates contemplative insight into the nature of reality. It is such insight that directly counteracts and eliminates self-grasping.

---

22. Translator's note: A clear, experiential account of contemplative means to eliminate self-grasping is presented in Gen Lamrimpa, *Realizing Emptiness: The Madhyamaka Cultivation of Insight*, trans. B. Alan Wallace (Ithaca: Snow Lion, 1999).

Chapter Six
The Accumulation, Arousal, and Pacification of Humoral Disorders

The explanation of the accumulation, arousal, and pacification of humoral disorders deals with (I) the causes, (II) the essential natures, and (III) the seasons for these phases of illness.[23]

The Causes

Food and medication having rough, light, subtle, hard, and motile qualities, when conjoined with the potency of warmth, cause wind to increase in its own locations, such as the bones, and wind disorders are thereby accumulated.[24] While the qualities of roughness and so on increase wind (due to their correspondence with the characteristics of wind), their conjunction with the potency of warmth suppresses wind, so the disorder cannot manifest. When those qualities of roughness and so on of one's food and medication are conjoined with the potency of coolness, wind disorders that have accumulated in their own location are aroused. The

---

23. These topics are discussed in *Bod kyi gso rig slob deb*, by Blo bzang bstan 'dzin (Dharamsala: Bod gzhung sman rtsis khang gso rig mtho slob sde tshan), Vol. I, pp. 284-289.

24. There are eight potencies derived from the five elements: heaviness and oiliness counteract wind disorders; coolness and dullness counteract bile disorders; and lightness, roughness, heat, and sharpness counteract phlegm disorders. *Bod rgya tshig mdzod chen mo* (Chengdu: Mi rigs dpe skrun khang, 1984), p. 1527.

unique combination of those qualities and that potency counteracts the suppression of wind disorders. Eventually, when wind disorders aroused by those causes are counteracted by food and medication having oily, warm, heavy, soft, and firm qualities, wind disorders are pacified in their own location.

Likewise, food and medication having sharp, oily, odorous,[25] purgative, and moist qualities, when conjoined with the potency of coolness, cause bile to increase in its own locations, such as the blood and sweat, and bile disorders are thereby accumulated. While the qualities of sharpness and so on increase bile (due to their correspondence with the characteristics of bile), their conjunction with the potency of coolness suppresses bile, so the disorder cannot manifest. When those qualities of sharpness and so on of one's food and medication are conjoined with the potency of heat, bile disorders that have accumulated in their own location are aroused. The unique combination of those qualities and that potency stop the suppression of bile disorders. Eventually, when bile disorders aroused by those causes are counteracted by food and medication having dull, dry, and cool qualities, bile disorders are pacified in their own location.

Similarly, food and medication having heavy, oily, dull, smooth, stable, and sticky qualities, when conjoined with the potency of coolness, cause phlegm to increase in its own locations, such as the nutriment, flesh and fat, and phlegm disorders are thereby accumulated. While the qualities of heaviness and so on increase phlegm (due to their correspondence with the characteristics of phlegm), their conjunction with the potency of coolness congeals and "freezes" phlegm, so the phlegm disorder cannot manifest. When those qualities of heaviness and so on of one's food and medication are conjoined with the potency of warmth, cool phlegm disorders that have accumulated in their own location are aroused. The unique combination of those qualities and that potency stops the containment of phlegm disorders. Eventually, when phlegm disorders aroused by those causes are counteracted by food and medication having rough, light, sharp, and motile qualities, phlegm disorders are pacified in their own location.

---

25. This quality (*dri mnam pa*) is both oily and moist.

The Essential Natures

Under the influences of one's diet, conduct, environment, and the seasons, wind, bile, and phlegm gradually increase in their own locations, and disorders are thereby accumulated. Due to those contributing conditions, the bodily constituents are disturbed and agitated, and one then craves food and drink having qualities opposite to those of the disturbed humors. For instance, when wind disorders are accumulated, one craves things having oily and heavy qualities and so on, which are the opposite of wind; likewise, when bile disorders are accumulated, one desires things having cool and dull qualities and so on; and when phlegm disorders are accumulated, one longs for things having light and rough qualities and so on. That is the essential nature of accumulation.

Under the influences of one's diet, conduct, environment, and the seasons, humoral disorders that have accumulated in their own locations enter other areas of the body, such as a wind disorder invading the locations of phlegm and bile. This gives rise to discomfort, and the individual symptoms of those disorders manifest in the pulse and urine. That is the essential nature of arousal.

By devoting oneself to a healthy diet, conduct, medical treatment, and environment, and due to the influence of the seasons, the humors are once again balanced in their own locations, and the symptoms of discomfort and so on disappear. That is the essential nature of pacification.

The Seasons

During the early summer (May-June), due to a light and rough environment, humoral constitution, diet, and conduct—all having similar characteristics—wind disorders are accumulated; but due to the warmth, they are not aroused. During the summer (July-August), they are aroused by rain, wind, and cold; and in the fall (September-October), they are pacified by the oiliness and warmth of that season. If wind-dominant people eat food and medicine having a bitter taste and light and rough potencies, and engage in light and rough conduct, due to the homogeneity of all those factors, wind increases in its own locations, and wind disorders are accumulated. However, due to the intense warmth of that season, the increase and accumulation of wind disorders are somewhat mitigated, or suppressed, so they are not aroused. But then under the influence of the coldness due to rain and wind during the late summer, the wind disorders accumulated in early summer are aroused in their own locations.

During the autumn, after the rain and wind of summer have ceased, and before the cold of winter has set in, the oily and warm potencies of that season—which are opposite to the characteristics of wind—pacify wind disorders in their own locations.

The qualities of the period July through August are oily and cool. As a result of this oily quality, bile increases; but the coolness of this season suppresses this increased bile, thereby preventing its arousal. This season is cool in India because this is the time of the monsoon. Then from September through October, the earlier potency of oiliness is retained, but the potency of warmth now arises, which allows for the arousal of the bile; and this can lead to an imbalance. Winter has the potency of coolness, and that naturally pacifies bile disorders.

Normally a bile disorder will be accumulated but not be aroused in the late summer. However, during the summer, if the region in which one dwells has dry, hot, and sharp potencies, and if one is young, this may arouse bile disorders. This is to say, there may be unseasonable weather during the late summer that is of a hot and sharp nature, and this would lead to the further accumulation of a bile disorder. This is all the more exacerbated if one's own constitution is of a predominately bile nature, and if one eats excessive amounts of hot and sour food and drink. Such an imbalance is all the more aggravated if one engages in violent, strenuous, or rough conduct.

Due to the confluence of all of these various factors, bile increases and an imbalance is accumulated. Why is this? Late summer (or monsoon) is a time when there is much wind and rain. The oiliness of this season allows for the increase of the bile, but the coolness suppresses, or conceals, that increase. When fall comes, with its oily, warm, and rough potencies, bile disorders naturally are aroused by those factors. During the fall, which is the season when a bile disorder is aroused and one feels ill, bile will be especially aroused at noon and midnight. If the bile disorder is not too serious, when the fall passes and winter comes, its cool and smooth qualities pacify the bile disorder and one recovers.

Late winter (January to February), with its cool, oily, heavy, and smooth potencies, acts to accumulate imbalances of the phlegm. Those four characteristics correspond to the primary characteristics of phlegm itself. However, those same qualities that allow it to accumulate also contain it, as if it had been put in the ice box. Then spring, with its warm potency, arrives, and this arouses phlegm disorders. With the advent of early summer, which is imbued with light and rough qualities, phlegm disorders are naturally pacified. In addition, if one is dwelling in a region that is wet and oily in late winter, such as the American south, and if one is a child and has a phlegmatic constitution, this will aggravate the accumulation of a phlegm disorder. Moreover, if one's diet consists largely of sweet, cool, and oily food and drink, and if one's conduct is phlegmatic, this will intensify the accumulation of phlegm disorders. As the result of all of those various factors coming together, phlegm disorders are accumulated but they are not aroused at that season. Why is that? Even though the characteristics of the region, one's diet, the season, and one's humoral constitution accumulate a phlegm disorder, due to the coolness of that period, it is as if the phlegm disorder is frozen, or immobilized and therefore cannot arise. However, when spring comes, with its warmth, it is as if the accumulated phlegm disorder thaws out, enabling it to arise. Then when early summer comes, with its light and rough qualities, the phlegm disorder naturally subsides and is pacified.

Although we may not notice these transitions, this is how our constitutions change from season to season. It is also possible for this process to speed up, occurring within a matter of a couple of days. For example, if one were to eat a lot of fatty foods one day, and the next day drank hard liquor, lay out in the sun, and engaged in strenuous exercise, this might give rise to a bile disorder, regardless of the season. To give a second example, if someone were to eat light and rough food, and then were to experience some anxiety, conflict, or fear, this might give rise to a wind disorder. To give a third example, if one were to ingest a lot of sweet fruit, drink large amounts of cold water, spend a good deal of time in cold water, and then wear light clothes and allow oneself to get cool, followed by heavy and oily diet, then, due to the confluence of these factors, a phlegm disorder might be aroused, regardless of the season. Thus, as a result of specific types of diet and behavior, disorders of the three humors may arise any time.

Chapter Seven
Conditions Contributing to Illness

Common Contributing Conditions of Illness

There are four conditions that may contribute to disorders, and these four are subdivided into the categories of common and specific conditions. Improper medical treatment is a common contributing factor for the occurrence of disease, and *karma* accumulated from previous lives is a special influence that may lead to illnesses arising in the body. To give an example of improper medical treatment, someone may have a bile disorder and accurately recognize it as such. One might then look at a Tibetan medical book that describes the efficacy of specific herbal compounds and find one that is said to alleviate bile disorders. Taking such medication may actually make one's illness worse. Even though this is a bile medication and one has a bile disorder, without knowing the specific qualities of the particular bile disorder, one will not know exactly which remedy, or combinations of remedies, will be helpful; and the wrong medication may actually aggravate the problem.

It is for similar reasons that in the West there are many medications that one cannot buy over the counter. Without knowing the precise efficacy of specific drugs, many of them could be dangerous, so in order to protect the consumer, such medicines must be prescribed by a physician. Likewise, in Tibetan medicine, it is important to be extremely cautious about choosing medications without having them prescribed by a skilled and experienced practitioner.

A new movement in the Tibetan medical tradition has occurred during my lifetime. Before I was born, there were a few texts in print that presented brief accounts of the efficacies of specific Tibetan medical compounds of herbs, minerals, and the like. This presented some danger for people who tried to diagnose themselves and choose their own remedies on the basis of these rough descriptions. Already when I was a youth in Tibet, however, new books were being composed that described the therapeutic efficacies of Tibetan medicines in much more elaborate detail, describing their specific potencies in terms of coolness, lightness, roughness and so on. They also gave detailed descriptions of the different types of humoral imbalances and indicated which medications are helpful for each kind of illness. Such works were helpful, so I believe that was a step in the right direction. Those textbooks have not been translated into Western languages. The material that has been translated thus far tends to be very sketchy, and this makes it more likely that if Westerners try to use them to diagnose and treat themselves on such a flimsy basis, they may well do themselves harm.

It is also possible that one may take a medication that initially was the right one, but if one continues taking that medicine as one gets better, it then makes one worse! That is, once the humors have been brought back into balance, one should not continue to take the medicine; otherwise, it may set up an imbalance all over again. That is another of the common contributing factors that may lead to disease. Taking too little of a medication may also be harmful, but generally that is not very problematic when taking herbal medication. If one takes too little, it is not likely to bring any harm.

Another of the common contributing factors is demonic influences. There are many types of non-human beings: demons, spirits, and the like. "Elemental" demonic forces called *bhūtas* may contribute to a number of infectious diseases. While such diseases are passed on from one person to another, they may also be reinforced by such demonic influences, which sustain the disease so that it cannot be cured by medication.

Generally speaking, a Tibetan physician needs to be aware of 404 different classes of disease, which are subdivided into 1616 (4 × 404) disorders. Among the 1616, one set of 101 consists of adventitious, relatively minor afflictions. These may be brought on by improper diet or conduct, and they will naturally heal by themselves. If one goes to a doctor and take medication for such a disease, it is like falling down and asking someone to lend a hand getting one back on one's feet—one could have done it with no assistance! A second set of the 101 diseases can be healed if proper medical treatment is given; otherwise, they are deadly. A third set of 101 consists of diseases that arise as a result of one's previous *karma* and generally result in death even if medical treatment is administered. However, if one does receive medical treatment and also applies oneself to virtue and spiritual purification of one's previous *karma,* it is possible to extend one's life span, even though the disease is not cured. A fourth set of 101 diseases consists of disorders inflicted by demonic influences. If one does not take additional action to expel or counteract such influences, medical treatment alone will not be effective; on the other hand, at times, methods to negate demonic influences may be effective even without medical treatment.

The situation has gotten a lot easier over the past couple of decades with the changes in Tibetan medical practice. When I was a child, Tibetan doctors commonly dispensed medication in powdered form, and they would give the patient a little round spoon with which to measure out the prescribed dosage of the herbal compound. But people would get sloppy, filling the spoon only halfway, over-filling it, or using another spoon altogether. In that way, they often took too much or too little of the medicine. But for some decades now, Tibetan doctors have generally formed medications in little pills, so that it is easy to take the proper amount.

Even if you have the medicine in pill form, how does one know whether one is taking it for too long or too short a period? Generally speaking, if you take it too short a time, it won't help you but it won't hurt either; and even if you take it too long, it won't likely do much harm. If you have a bile disorder and take too much bile medication, that could do some damage, but if you take medicine for a wind disorder longer than needed, it will just calm you down further. In the case of phlegm disorders, you generally have to take medication for a long time anyway, because such disorders are sluggish and do not mend swiftly.

For example, there are various types of tumors, including cancerous ones, that are related to wind, bile, and phlegm. If a tumor is affiliated with a bile disorder, it grows quite quickly; if it is associated with a wind disorder, it will alternatingly grow and then go into remission; and if it is affiliated with a phlegm disorder, it will grow very slowly and have few symptoms. The paucity of symptoms of a phlegm-related tumor is not necessarily a bad thing. In fact, among the tumors, those are the best type to have, for they are relatively easy to treat either with surgery or with herbal medications. The dangerous ones are those affiliated with wind and bile disorders. Those associated with bile disorders are the worst, because they grow large very quickly, and even if they are surgically removed, since they are of the nature of the bile—aggressive, arrogant, and fast-moving—such tumors may quickly spread from one region of the body to another.

In modern medical textbooks composed in Tibet under Chinese Communist rule, a great deal of information is synthesized in a single text. This new mode of presentation is, I believe, harmful for students who are taking the full course of training in Tibetan medicine, for this could lead them to believe that the traditional treatises are obsolete or irrelevant. However, this approach is useful to provide a general introduction to this medical system, and in this sense it is good for initially presenting this material in the West. We have the Chinese Communists to thank for this. What they have done is synthesize the material from many traditional Tibetan medical texts, and they have excised all the references to the spiritual aspects of this tradition. Thus, they deal only with the purely physical aspects of the body, health, disease, and so forth, while leaving out all the spiritual depth and ramifications of this discipline.

A distant relative of mine named Kunga Phuntsok is very highly placed in the Tibetan Medical Center in Lhasa. In the late 1970s and during the 1980s, he visited me in India and described to me how colleagues of his are composing these new books based upon the earlier ones, and he showed me examples of their work. He found that the authors of these new texts are scrambling up the traditional presentations of *The Four Tantras,* and he told the authors that perhaps this was suitable for the young people in Tibet, but he did not feel they were open to any advice or criticisms he might have to give. I feel the people doing this are really transforming the whole tradition of Tibetan medicine, as if they were continuing the trends promoted during the Cultural Revolution. The last time he visited me was in 1989, when he showed me some of their recent compositions. The justification for creating these new textbooks was that the young students in Tibet today refuse to study the traditional treatises; so they must teach them modern works on the subject. In response, he just smiled, because he knew it really was out of his hands.

Kunga Phuntsok is an elderly man, and he was not advocating this change; rather, he was witnessing something that was beyond his control. In fact, he was hoping that he could somewhat stem the tide of these changes, and return to the more traditional ways of teaching, but he recognized he could not be successful in this pursuit. These doctors in Tibet under Chinese Communist domination are actually mimicking modern Western traditions. In the traditional training in Tibetan medicine, all students master all *The Four Tantras,* and no one specializes in specific body parts such as the ears, nose, mouth, and so on. Tibetan medicine is essentially a holistic system, so one must understand all the interrelationships among the organs and other body parts. But now, with the advent of these new textbooks and methods of education, Tibetan medical students, like Western interns, are being trained in specialities within this medical tradition, such as diseases of the eyes, ears, nose and so on. This approach is antithetical to the spirit of Tibetan medicine as a whole. Kunga Phuntsok has been caught between these two worlds, and he has been disheartened with these changes.

Specific Contributing Conditions

The specific conditions that contribute to disorders of the wind humor include ingesting medication, food or drink that taste bitter and light and that have rough, motile, hard, thin, dry (i.e., non-oily), or cold potencies. Other conditions specifically leading to wind imbalances include frustration, grief, melancholy, tempestuous emotions including misery, intense craving, inadequate food and sleep, strenuous physical activity (especially on an empty stomach), and excessive conversation. Loss of blood due to such things as a nosebleed or a wound, diarrhea, violent vomiting, forcefully restraining one's bowels, urine, and sneezing, using excessive force to defecate or urinate, and remaining in a cool, windy place may also contribute to wind disorders.

The specific conditions that contribute to bile disorders include ingesting food that is spicy, hot, sharp, or oily, experiencing strong hatred or anger, sleeping excessively during the daytime, and immediately thereafter engaging in vigorous activity, such as carrying heavy objects, using a pick-axe to break very hard ground, drawing bows with very high tension, swimming, running, or riding and falling off horses. Falling off precipices, being buried under rubble from a collapsed house and so forth, being physically beaten, and eating too much butter, raw sugar or meat followed by drinking soft and hard liquor are also contributing conditions that may lead to a bile disorder.

The conditions that contribute to phlegm disorders include ingesting too much sweet, bitter, heavy, oily, and cool food and drink, and then lounging around or falling asleep. Moreover, if one sleeps on moist earth or wet grass, the moisture will rise up and contribute to a phlegm disorder, but this does not happen if one is on a lounge chair or on a rubber or leather mat. A phlegm disorder may also be aroused if one spends a lot of time in cold water and then dresses scantily and eats uncooked or unripe corn or beans, which have a cold quality. Once they fully ripen, the result is different. Other contributing conditions include ingesting goat meat, fat or raw meat, oil produced from grains or other substances, cow and sheep butter, stale or rotten food, raw vegetables (especially turnips and carrots), and raw mountain-grown garlic. If those foods are not cooked sufficiently or are burnt, that can also lead to phlegm disorders. Cold-cuts, stale milk, and yogurt from goats, sheep, or cows, low-fat yogurt, and excessive eating or drinking such that one begins eating before having digested the food already consumed are further conditions that may lead to a phlegm disorder.

Chapter Eight

The Manners of Entrance of Illnesses

The causes and conditions leading to diseases are like drawing an arrow on a bow. Once the three poisons of attachment, hatred, and delusion have arisen as the primary causes of the disease and have conjoined with the necessary contributing factors for a disease to occur, the targets to which the disease is now propelled like an arrow are wind, bile, and phlegm. The archer is analogous to the contributing conditions, including the seasons, demonic influences, and diet and conduct. Once those factors have infiltrated the body and have produced an imbalance of the humors, that disruption leads to other maladies where the various humors are located. Briefly stated, wind disorders are generally located in the bones; bile disorders are located in the blood, bile, and sweat; and phlegm disorders are located in the remaining bodily constituents, namely, the flesh, nutriment, fat, bone marrow, regenerative substances, excrement, and urine. We need to be aware of the interactions among all these constituents of the body. For example, a disorder of the life-sustaining wind could lead to an imbalance of the decomposing phlegm, which could impair the digestive bile, and that, in turn, could impair the fire-accompanying wind.

The six entrances through which the illnesses come into the body are the following: Illnesses first spread on the skin, then expand through the flesh, move through the channels, cling to the bone, descend upon the solid organs (the heart, lungs, kidneys, liver, and spleen), and fall upon the hollow organs (the stomach, gall bladder, small intestine, urinary bladder, the vesicles of the regenerative substances, and the large intestine).

Wind disorders are located in the pelvis, the joints, and the skin (where one feels tactile sensations), the ears, and the large intestine (specifically the ascending transverse colon). Those are where symptoms of wind disorders are experienced. Among those areas, the principal location of wind disorders is the large intestine.

The principal locations of bile disorders and their symptoms are in the small intestine, the blood, sweat, nutriment, serous fluid, eyes, and the skin; and among those regions bile disorders are located principally in the area of the small intestine, in which the food is digested, and that is where one experiences such illnesses. As in the case of wind disorders, the actual symptoms of bile disorders are experienced in these regions. Bile disorders in the skin manifest differently than wind disorders of the skin. Bile disorders of the skin include the symptoms of itching and redness, which are related to one's lymphatic system. In contrast, if a wind disorder manifests in the skin, this results in numbness and insensitivity to cold and heat. When the body is in a state of balance, the color-transforming bile located in the skin gives one a clear, healthy complexion. However, when this bile is in a state of disorder, it leads to itching and so forth.

The locations of the phlegm disorders are the chest, throat, lungs, and the head. Such disorders are pervasive. They reside in the nutriment before the production of blood, but not in the blood itself. In addition, they are located in the flesh, fat, marrow, regenerative substances, urine, excrement, nose, tongue, and in the stomach, where the food is yet to be digested. As in the previous two cases, the actual symptoms of phlegm disorders are experienced in those locations where the phlegm disorder is present.

Chapter Nine

The Characteristics of Humoral Imbalances

I will now explain the characteristics of the humors when they are in a state of imbalance. There are three ways in which the humors may be imbalanced: a state of excess, deficiency, or disturbance. These three categories of imbalances are applied to the ten afflicted elements, namely, the seven bodily constituents and the three waste products. To understand the states of excess, deficiency, and disturbance of the three humors, one must understand these three conditions in relation to the seven bodily constituents, the three waste products, and the fifteen sub-classes of wind, bile and phlegm. But for simplicity's sake I shall now address the causes and symptoms of the ten afflicted elements only.

The conditions of deficiency and excess are relative to the appropriate quantities of the ten afflicted elements. I shall first discuss the causes of an excess and a deficiency of the humors. The first cause of such an excess or deficiency is an unhealthy diet and conduct. Dietary causes of an excess of the wind humor include insufficient meat, alcohol, and sweet food or drink, too little food, and over-consumption of light and rough food and drink. Behavioral causes include becoming chilled, engaging in excessively strenuous activity, and participating in disagreeable types of activities. If one persists in those types of diet and conduct, the wind increases to a state of excess.

Over-consumption of oily, fatty foods and rich foods gives rise to an excess of bile; and if one persists in that, eventually one's complexion turns yellowish. Over-consumption of heavy, oily, and sticky food results in an excess of phlegm.

Symptoms of Excess

Symptoms of an excess of wind include weight loss, darkening of the complexion, craving for warmth, chills and shivering, abdominal distention due to gas, difficulty in defecating, loquaciousness, dizziness as if intoxicated, decline of physical strength, insomnia, and loss of clarity in one's sense faculties and intelligence. Symptoms of an excess of bile include a yellowish tinge in the excrement, urine, skin, and the sclera of the eyes, strong hunger and thirst, excessive bodily heat, inability to sleep sufficiently, and looseness of the bowels (to the point of diarrhea). Symptoms of an excess of phlegm include a decrease in warmth throughout the body, poor digestion, abdominal distention due not to gas but to phlegm[26] (which can lead to stomach acidity, and that, in turn, may lead to ulcers), heaviness of the body, lethargy, pale complexion, flaccidity of the limbs, excessive accumulation of thick saliva in the mouth, excessive sputum, heavy sleep, and difficulty in breathing. The Tibetan medical tradition lists five types of asthma, and the principal one entails an excess of phlegm. All types of asthma are fundamentally phlegm disorders, but among them there is a fivefold classification. There are types of asthma that entail phlegm and bile, phlegm and blood, and phlegm and lymph, and so forth. This type of imbalance is located in the lungs, and its symptoms include sneezing and difficulty in respiration.

Moving now to the bodily constituents, the symptoms of an excess of the nutriment are identical to those for an excess of phlegm, so there is a danger of confusing these two. One symptom of an excess of the blood is a rash consisting of round, itchy blotches of various sizes all over the skin, and the skin around them is very rough. According to popular Tibetan lore (not the textual medical tradition), if these blotches form a ring around the neck, this is a sign that one will die. These blotches are red, a little darker in the center, and the flesh around them is raw and uneven. Another symptom of an excess of blood is the formation of growths (*'bras*) in the stomach and small intestine. Such growths can be surgically removed, but they tend to reappear. All spleen disorders, all types of leprosy, blood and bile disorders, and most but not all types of tumors come from an excess of the blood. In the case of such an excess,

---

26. This can lead to stomach acidity, and if left untreated, that may result in the formation of ulcers. This occurs when such an imbalance is "accumulated" and manifests, and one does not take proper medication to alleviate it.

the eyes become yellow, and the skin just above the eyes, the eyelids, and the gums become swollen and red.

Symptoms of an excess of flesh include goiters and the occurrence of cysts, or nodular masses (e.g., subcutaneous nodules, dermal cysts, and lipomas), on the skin under the armpits, behind the ears, in the throat, in the groin, and the lower abdomen above the hips. Most of the mass of these firm growths is beneath the skin, but they do protrude somewhat against the skin. If these occur on the limbs or on the back, they are not serious, but those that occur on the throat, behind the ears, under the armpits, in the groin or the lower abdomen may be dangerous. Cysts are commonly surgically removed in the West for fear that they may lead to cancer, but this may have harmful effects. If these cysts are due to an excess of bile and are surgically removed, that may help; but if they are due to an excess of wind, that may exacerbate the problem because wind causes them to spread quickly, so they may proliferate. When these cysts are exacerbated, they lead to lymphoma. According to Tibetan medicine, the disease identified as lymphoma in the Western tradition may be of two types: one pertains to these enlarged cysts and the other is in fact a disturbance of the blood.

Symptoms of an excess of the fat include exhaustion, lethargy, and anemia (which can be mistaken for hypoglycemia). In addition, the body becomes heavy, one becomes dazed, one's intelligence becomes dull, and whether one is a man or a woman, the breasts become large and the abdomen protrudes.

Symptoms of an excess of the bone include the formation of bone spurs and excess teeth. Symptoms of an excess of bone marrow include a feeling of heaviness of the body and poor vision. Symptoms of an excess of the regenerative substances include the formation of stones in the kidneys, the urinary bladder, and the urinary tract, and an increase of one's libido, or sexual drive.

As for the waste products, the symptoms of an excess of the excrement include a feeling of heaviness in the body, abdominal bloating, morgarigamy (abdominal gurgling), and bodily stiffness, making movement difficult. Symptoms of an excess of urine are shooting pains in the urinary tract and a feeling that one has not urinated, even though one has done so. Symptoms of an excess of sweat include a pungent and disagreeable odor to the body whenever sweat is exuded, and itching (even in the absence of any kind of rash or pimples).

Symptoms of Deficiency

I shall now describe the symptoms of a deficiency of the individual humors and bodily constituents. If the wind is deficient, one has little energy for any kind of task, one feels disinclined to talk, and one becomes disengaged from, or out of touch with, one's own emotions. For example, one may be happy without being particularly aware of it. With such a deficiency, the clarity of one's mindfulness and memory declines. Note the virtual equivalence of the symptoms of an excess of phlegm and a deficiency of wind. The only difference is that with a wind deficiency one does not feel like talking, whereas this is not a symptom of an excess of phlegm.

The symptoms of a deficiency of bile include a decrease in the warmth of the body and the luster of the skin, one feels cold, and one's complexion becomes dark.

If the phlegm is deficient, the body cannot properly produce nutriment, which gradually leads to weight loss. It is very easy to mistake a deficiency of phlegm for an excess of wind, but they are not the same. The elements associated with phlegm are water and earth, and when these elements in the brain diminish, this impairs the functioning of the phlegm in the brain, resulting in dizziness and palpitation of the heart. Specifically due to a depletion of the connective phlegm, all the joints feel loose or slack, for it is the connective phlegm that keeps them firm.

Moving now to each of the seven bodily constituents, symptoms of a deficiency of the nutriment include weight loss and difficulty in swallowing. The skin takes on a coarse, rough texture, and one becomes very sensitive to loud noises. These symptoms appear like those of a wind disorder, but the underlying illness is different.

A symptom of a deficiency of blood is that one's channels become loose, meaning that when analyzing the pulse, the blood veins do not feel firm to the touch. Rather, they feel flaccid, as if they are empty, and the veins near the surface of the skin do not protrude as usual, but seem to sink into the flesh as if they were empty. In addition, one's skin takes on a rough texture, and a decrease in the warmth of the blood leads to a coolness of the body.

The symptoms of a deficiency of the flesh are discomfort in the joints as if one had been beaten, weight loss, and a feeling as if one's skin were adhering to the bones.

The symptoms of a deficiency of fat are that one sleeps little, and the body becomes thin and takes on a bluish complexion.

Symptoms of a deficiency of bone include hair loss, degeneration of the teeth so that they are prone to breaking or falling out, and stunted and crooked growth of the nails.

Symptoms of a deficiency of bone marrow include a sensation of hollowness inside the bones, as if they were filled with air, dizziness, and a "veiling of the eyesight." Such veiling, or dimming, of the eyes occurs when one is afflicted with diabetes.

The symptoms of a deficiency of the regenerative substances pertain only to the semen, for the female regenerative substance is never deficient, not even after menopause. When the semen is deficient, one ejaculates blood instead of semen, sexual enjoyment decreases, and one experiences a hot, burning sensation in the urinary tract, the urinary bladder, and the testicles.

Moving now to the waste products, symptoms of a deficiency of excrement include morgarigamy and a sensation as if the abdomen is filled with air, and this can lead to palpitations of the heart. This entails brief, intermittent periods of discomfort in the heart, the ribcage, and the sternum.

Symptoms of a deficiency of urine include discoloration, dysuria, and urinating in small amounts at a time.

Symptoms of a deficiency of sweat are cracks in the skin, and one's body hair stands on end and is prone to falling out. When there is a deficiency of any of the minor waste products, such as the excretions from the nose, eyes, and ears, there is discomfort in those respective places. When each of the bodily constituents is in balance—when each of them is functioning properly in its own place and in relationship to others—then the three waste products remain in balance; that is, they are not in excess, not deficient, and not disturbed.

The most refined nutriment that is located in the life-force channel behind the heart may be depleted due to intense grief, trauma, or anxiety, and the symptoms of such a deficiency are frequent anxiety, fear, and even terror, a general deterioration of one's health, loss of weight, vitality, and strength, emotional frailty, and loss of interest and enjoyment in all types of activities including work and play. One feels apathetic toward everything, and the splendor of the body also declines. To remedy such a deficiency one should take medication from a qualified Tibetan doctor. It helps to eat sweet food, highly nutritious food, and vital essence pills,

which are a kind of super tonic. In addition, one should ingest an aphro-
disiac to increase one's libido, freshly milked sheep or cow milk before it
loses its warmth from the udder, meat juice, and other tonics that may
be prescribed by one's doctor. This very refined nutriment is the basis for
one's longevity and vitality, so by remedying a deficiency of that nutriment, one's life span will be increased.

Symptoms of Disturbance

The symptoms of disturbance pertain only to the three humors, and I
shall first address common symptoms of wind disturbances. One symptom of such a disturbance is an "empty, fluctuating pulse," meaning that
when one first examines the pulse, it is clearly detected, but then it seems
to disappear, or become "empty." Another symptom is that as soon as
one urinates, while it is still warm, the urine is clear like mountain spring
water, and then it becomes even more limpid as it cools off.

There are nine features to examine when performing urine analysis.
When the urine is still hot, one examines its (1) color, (2) vapor, (3)
odor, and (4) froth. Then when the urine has cooled off somewhat, when
it is still lukewarm, one examines (5) the suspended sediment, or cloudi-
ness, in the urine, and (6) the oily skim, or chyle, on the surface. Finally,
when the urine is cold, one examines (7) the gradations of coloring of
the urine, (8) the ways in which the color of the urine changes while it is
cooling, and (9) the final color of the urine after it has cooled off completely. The many gradations of coloration of the urine pertain to the
wind, bile, phlegm, dual combinations, and threefold combinations of
the humors. Each of these has its own specific patterns of coloration,
from top to bottom, and from the middle to the periphery. This is a
complex topic, which would take about twenty days to explain completely. Moreover, by examining these specific patterns, one can determine if there are any kinds of demonic influences harming the patient.

In the case of a wind disturbance, there is little odor or vapor from the
urine, and the bubbles of the froth are large "like buffalo eyeballs." The
final color of the urine after it has cooled down is bluish, as it was when
it was first discharged, which means that it is clear and limpid like mountain spring water.

Due to the motile nature of the wind humor, the symptoms of such a
disorder are intermittent, and they move around in the body. One tends
to be exhausted and sigh frequently, even if one has not worked very

hard. The mind also becomes unstable as in cases of attention deficit disorders, for one cannot focus on anything for very long. In addition, one may experience dizziness and at times even faint, although this is generally not associated with seizures. One may hear roaring in the ears, and one's hearing may be impaired. The tongue becomes dry, red, and rough, and one does not taste one's food very distinctly. Moreover, the food one eats may seem to have an astringent quality.

One may experience shooting pains and other types of discomfort that rove about in the body without remaining in any one place for long. Such sporadic discomfort, including itching, may be especially in the hips or arms. One may experience occasional chills, shivering, goose bumps, and muscular twitches in various parts of the body. Wind disorders are located in areas where one has tactile sensations, so this refers not only to the skin but anywhere tactile sensations are experienced. With a wind disturbance, one may be subject to absentmindedness and forgetfulness. For example, one may intend to perform a certain task, but when the time comes to do it, one has forgotten all about it. The body seems to be light but stiff, and it may feel crooked, stooped, and uncomfortable. There is a sensation as if one's skin has come detached from the flesh, and one may feel as if the bones and joints are broken, and the joints hurt and feel as if they are unhinged.

All of one's sensory faculties have a constricted quality. The eyes feel tight and constricted, as does the whole body, as though it were bound up. When one moves the body, it feels painful all over. One may experience insomnia during the nighttime, and during the day there may be excessive yawning, and the body may be prone to shaking and trembling. One feels like stretching again and again. One becomes irritable and is easily upset. There may be special discomfort in the hip joints and the femur as if they had been beaten with a club, as well as the back, especially around the sixth and the seventh cervical vertebrae. The jawbones also hurt, and one may feel nauseous and experience dry heaves, throwing up nothing more than froth. In addition, there may be abdominal distention and morgarigamy. Swellings and tumors that grow as a result of a wind disturbance fluctuate in size, appearing in one place and then vanishing. The symptoms of wind disturbances are especially evident in the evening, at dawn, and after one has digested food.

Moving now to the common symptoms of a bile disturbance, the pulse is overflowing in the sense that when one detects it, there is a sense of fullness. The pulse is also thin, fast, and taut, like a tight string on a guitar. As for the characteristics of the urine, it is orange, malodorous, and has a lot of vapor. When the urine is agitated, its froth consists of small bubbles that form and vanish quickly.

Other symptoms of a bile disturbance include headaches, excessive heat in the body, and a sour taste in the mouth. The tongue feels thick, and it is covered with a film of light yellow phlegm, which is sticky like glue. The nostrils are dry, and the sclera become yellow. Wherever pain arises in the body as a result of the disturbance of the bile, it stays there. It does not rove around, as in the case of a wind disturbance. In the evening, one sleeps very little, but in the afternoon it is very hard to stay awake. When one coughs, one coughs up an orangish spittle with bubbles in it of the same color. One's own saliva may taste salty, bitter, or sour, though bitterness is the most common taste. One tends to be thirsty, and because of the disturbance of bile and blood, one is prone to both diarrhea and vomiting. If one suffers from loose bowels or diarrhea, one may pass bile and blood in the stool. If one vomits, blood and bile may also appear in the vomit, and it has a very bitter taste. One's sweat becomes malodorous, and the stool has an orangish color and is also malodorous and putrid.

One's facial complexion, as well as the color of the teeth take on an orangish tinge. Swelling and all types of tumors that occur as a result of a bile disturbance tend to grow very quickly. If they occur on or near the surface of the skin, they will rapidly emerge through the skin, producing pus. If a tumor forms in the lungs, it also produces pus, which may emerge from the mouth, but with no external symptoms on the skin. If a tumor occurs inside the throat, pus is also produced and comes out the mouth. Boils that are due to a bile disturbance tend to grow very quickly, burst, and then produce pus. The symptoms of a bile disturbance are especially strong at noon, at midnight, and while food is being digested.

Among the symptoms of a phlegm disturbance, the pulse is "sunken" or "dull," which is to say that it is weak, slow, and hard to detect. For the sake of clarification, the pulse of the body when it is in a balanced state beats five times during each of the physician's inhalations and exhalations. Here is the general rule of thumb: If there are more than five pulse beats during the exhalation and inhalation of the physician, this indicates a heat disorder. If there are fewer than five pulse beats during a full respiration of the physician, that indicates a cold disorder.

In the case of a phlegm disturbance, the urine is pale in color, with little odor or vapor, and the froth on the urine is soft like the froth of saliva. Because of the malfunction of the experiencing phlegm, one cannot detect tastes clearly. The gums and tongue become pale, the sclera turn white and lackluster. The face becomes a little swollen. The mucus in the nose and the mouth increase. One becomes dazed as if suddenly finding oneself in an alien place. The body and mind feel heavy, and one experiences a loss of appetite. There is little warmth in the body, and one's digestion is impaired. There may be discomfort in the pelvis and the kidneys, and one has a feeling as if the body were swollen or bloated. A phlegm disturbance may produce goiters, and due to the malfunctioning of the decomposing phlegm, after ingesting food or drink, one spits it up again. Or, if the ascending wind does not cause one to spit it up, the descending wind will excrete them as waste products when they are still undigested. One's mindfulness, memory, and vision become unclear. One becomes lethargic, apathetic, and sluggish throughout the day and night. There may be itching on the skin even though there is no rash or pimples. Because of the malfunction of the connective phlegm, one has a feeling of stiffness in both the major and minor limbs, including the toes, fingers, arms, hands, legs, and so on. It becomes difficult to extend and retract one's limbs because they feel stiff. In addition, one becomes prone to obesity. These symptoms come especially at dusk, in the morning, and as soon as one has eaten.

This concludes the discussion of the symptoms of an excess, deficiency, and disturbance of the various constituents of the body. All types of disorders are included in those categories. The symptoms of an excess, deficiency, and disturbance of any twofold or threefold combination of the humors can be inferred upon the basis of the preceding discussion. A disturbance of just one humor is very rare. Understanding the symptoms related to the excess, deficiency, and disturbance of the three humors sheds light on all types of disorders.

Chapter Ten
Classifications of Diseases

Classifications of diseases are made on the basis of their (I) causes, (II) the body types in which they manifest, and (III) the characteristics of the disorders themselves.

The Classification of Diseases on the Basis of Their Causes

The classification of illnesses on the basis of their causes pertains to the three poisons of the mind—attachment, hatred and delusion—which are the fundamental causes of all diseases. In general, illnesses are brought about by factors in this life, in conjunction with one's *karma* accumulated from previous lifetimes. More precisely, one can speak of illnesses caused by three types of causes: (A) causes in this lifetime, (B) *karma* accumulated in previous lifetimes, and (C) a confluence of factors in this lifetime in conjunction with *karma* accumulated in previous lifetimes.

(A) There are two types of factors in this lifetime, (1) internal and (2) external, that may lead to disease.

(1) The internal causes consist of disturbance of the three humors, which are naturally present in the body. The manner in which these three humors act as causes of illness has already been discussed in terms of their excess, deficiency, and disturbance. These are the primary causes of illness in this lifetime.

(2) Within this lifetime there are adventitious, external conditions that may lead to illness, of which there are three kinds: (a) poisons, (b) weapons, such as spears, swords, stones, poison-tipped arrows, and in the modern world all manner of new chemical, biological, and nuclear weapons, and (c) demonic influences.

(B) The second of the three types of causes is *karma* from such deeds as the ten nonvirtues of killing and so forth. Three of those ten nonvirtues (killing, stealing, and sexual misconduct) pertain to the body, four to the speech (lying, slander, abuse, and idle gossip), and three to the mind (avarice, malice, and holding false views). Thus, the maturation of any type of nonvirtuous *karma,* or deed, from any previous lives is the second of these three types of causes.

(C) The third type of cause entails a conjunction of factors in this lifetime and one's previous *karma.* Specifically, the three humors in this lifetime are affected by the maturation of nonvirtues from previous lives, especially the ten nonvirtues.

In general, there are four factors in this life that may contribute to diseases: (1) the seasons, (2) demonic influences, (3) diet, and (4) conduct. Moreover, it often happens that a small cause has a major impact on one's health. For example, a minor disorder may be influenced by other circumstances and thus lead to very serious health problems. One cannot always fully account for this effect on the basis of the above four factors. When this happens, we conclude there must be some influence from *karma* that has been accumulated in previous lifetimes.

Demonic influences include a wide variety of influences from nonhuman agencies, including the planets, *devas, yaksas,*[27] *bhūtas,*[28] *nāgas,*[29] *pārthivas,*[30] and *ksamāpatis.*[31] According to the Tibetan medical tradition, *nāgas* and *ksamāpatis* frequently contribute to the formation of various types of tumors. In such cases in traditional Tibet, first offerings and propitiatory rituals would be made with respect to these entities. Once

---

27. Translator's note: Tib. *gnod sbyin.* A type of powerful being who may be called upon to aid one in one's spiritual practice, but who may also cause one physical harm.

28. Translator's note: Tib. *'byung po.* "Elemental" demonic forces, of which there are 1,080 types.

29. Translator's note: Tib. *klu.* Serpentlike creatures, many of whom dwell in bodies of water such as rivers and lakes. From an esoteric perspective, their actual nature is that of delusions produced by the causes and conditions of ignorance.

30. Translator's note: Tib. *rgyal po.* Demonic forces that emerge due to grasping onto the *I;* in reality they consist of the conceptual mental factors that reify appearances. Such beings are created by conceptually focusing on them, and they arise as apparitions of hatred.

31. Translator's note: Tib. *sa bdag.* Earth spirits, whose actual nature is that of delusions produced by the causes and conditions of ignorance.

this was done, medication would be given, and the combination of these methods often effected a cure.

In addition, there are another 360 types of entities which may possess an individual and thereby alter the mind and personality traits. A lot of mental disorders are attributed, at least in part, to the influence of such entities. In many cases of mental imbalances, there are specific ways of identifying which among these different types of non-human agencies may be responsible. A skilled Tibetan doctor is able to identify specifically which type of non-human agency is responsible for a specific disorder based upon the conduct and other symptoms of the patient. This is a very complex topic, but in the modern West, there is little point in discussing such non-human influences, for few people believe in their existence. This concludes the discussion of the classifications of diseases in terms of their causes.

The Classification of Diseases on the Basis of Body Types

Within this second classification, there is a fivefold subclassification of disorders of men, women, children, old people, and disorders common to everyone.

The illnesses to which men alone are prone include (1) a deficiency of semen, (2) an "excess of semen," which refers to an overactive libido, and (3-8) six diseases entailing swelling of the testicles, and nine diseases of the male genital organ.[32] These disorders may arise due to the six factors of (9) wind, (10) bile, (11) phlegm, (12) a blood disorder, (13) a combined disorder of wind, bile, and phlegm, and (14) the formation of boils and pustules on the genital organ. (15) Another male disorder, which seems to occur fairly commonly in America, is one in which the blood veins in the penis become knotted. This can occur in the flesh inside the penis or on the surface, and it is very painful. (16) Another illness entails a contraction of the urinary tract itself, which involves swelling and contraction, so it is very difficult for urine to pass along that canal. (17) The final disorder entails a very painful burning sensation in the testicles and the penis, as if they are on fire. The preceding illnesses may arise due to wind, bile, phlegm, and blood, or due to a combination of any of the preceding.

---

32. One of these entails the formation of pustules in the male urinary tract. If these pustules appear on the tip of the penis, that is not serious, but when they occur inside the urinary tract, this can be dangerous.

Among women's illnesses, there are five disorders of the ovaries, the uterus, and the breasts, which arise due to (1) wind, (2) bile, (3) phlegm, (4) blood, or from (5) a combination of any of those four. There are (6-14) nine types of tumors that may form in the ovaries, uterus, or the breasts, but I shall discuss these in detail in my explanation of benign and malignant tumors. Women are prone to (15-16) two types of diseases of the uterus caused by microorganisms. These microorganisms play a role in the activation of the woman's libido: when woman's libido is also aroused, these minute organisms are aroused, and improper conduct by a woman disturbs these organisms. Finally, there are (17-32) sixteen types of women's disorders related to the menstrual blood.

In addition, there are twenty-four types of children's diseases and other diseases of old people.[33] Finally, the diseases common to everyone include (1) 101 disorders caused by the humors, (2) 101 principal humoral disorders, (3) 101 disorders according to location, and (4) 101 disorders according to type.[34]

Diseases Common to Everyone

1. Disorders Caused by the Humors

Among the disorders caused by the humors, the general wind disorders include (1-20) twenty wind imbalances, (21-26) six types of wind disorders based on their paths of entry,[35] (27) wind disorders pertaining to the five sensory organs, (28-32) five disorders caused by the five types of wind, and (33-42) ten disorders caused by wind in conjunction with the five types of bile and the five types of phlegm. There are twenty-six general and specific bile disorders, and thirty-three diseases caused by phlegm. That comes to a total of 101 disorders caused by the humors.

Within one class of 404 diseases, the first set of 101 diseases includes the above humoral disorders when they are caused by temporary circumstances, such as becoming chilled, eating unhealthy food, and so

---

33. Translator's note: These are cited in *The Quintessence Tantras of Tibetan Medicine*, trans. Dr. Barry Clark (Ithaca: Snow Lion, 1995), p. 89.

34. Translator's note: This final set of 101 disorders, not explained in this volume, is discussed in the *Encyclopedia of Tibetan Medicine*, Vaidya Bhagwan Dash (Delhi: Sri Satguru Publications, 1994), Vol. II, pp. 171-181.

35. These include (1) penetrating the skin, (2) expanding in the flesh, (3) moving through the channels, (4) settling in the bones, (5) descending on the solid organs, and (6) falling on the hollow organs.

forth. Another set of 101 diseases includes those humoral disorders when they are brought about by actions committed in this life, and a third set of 101 diseases includes those humoral disorders due to *karma* accumulated in past lifetimes. The fourth set of 101 diseases includes those humoral disorders when they are due to demonic influences.

2. Principal Humoral Disorders

Principal humoral disorders may be either simple or complex. Simple humoral imbalances entail only one humor, whereas complex humoral imbalances involve a combination of two or more humors. In addition, there are subclassifications of great and extreme excess and deficiency of the humors.

Within the class of simple humoral imbalances, for (1) wind, (2) bile, and (3) phlegm disorders, there is the threefold classification of (a) general, (b) great, and (c) extreme (i) excess and (ii) deficiency, making a total of eighteen classes of humoral imbalances.

Within the class of complex disorders, there are combinations of two and three humoral imbalances. For example, there may be an imbalance of wind and bile, for which one prescribes medication to balance the wind, but which may, by itself, exacerbate the bile disorder. Likewise, medicine for a bile disorder may, by itself, exacerbate a wind disorder, so these two types of treatment must counteract each other's possible detrimental effects. To give an analogy, if you are talking to two people, while you are talking to one, the other may become exasperated. You are in a situation in which you cannot please both of them at the same time. Complex disorders can also involve three humors, which makes treatment all the more complex, so diseases of this kind are very difficult to treat.

Among complex disorders, there may be an equal excess of (1) wind and bile, (2) bile and phlegm, or (3) wind and phlegm. A further classification refers to unequal excess. For example, there may be (4) a great excess of wind and an extreme excess of bile, (5) a great excess of wind and an extreme excess of phlegm, (6) a great excess of phlegm and an extreme excess of bile, (7) a great excess of phlegm and an extreme excess of wind, (8) a great excess of bile and an extreme excess of wind, (9) and a great excess of bile and an extreme excess of phlegm. That makes a total of nine types of humoral imbalances of excess.

As for imbalances of deficiency, there may be an equal deficiency of (1) wind and bile, (2) phlegm and bile, and (3) phlegm and wind. When one includes the six further classifications of unequal deficiencies as above, this makes a total of eighteen complex humoral imbalances of deficiency.

As for threefold humoral disorders, the first classification includes an equal excess of all three humors. Other permutations include an extreme excess of wind, a great excess of bile, and a general excess of phlegm; an extreme excess of wind, a great excess of phlegm, and a general excess of bile. Similar permutations can be made for phlegm and bile, making a total of six permutations. Then there may be a general excess of wind and a great excess of both phlegm and bile; a general excess of bile and a great excess of phlegm and wind; and a great excess of phlegm and an extreme excess of wind and bile. A further permutation is of a general excess of wind and bile and a great excess of phlegm; a general excess of phlegm and bile and a great excess of wind; and a general excess of phlegm and wind and a great excess of the bile, which yields another six permutations. All those permutations can then be listed in reverse order and also applied to the varying degrees of both excess and deficiency. This would include the permutations of an extreme deficiency of wind, a great deficiency of bile, and a general deficiency of phlegm; an extreme deficiency of wind, a great deficiency of phlegm, and a general deficiency of bile. The same permutations are then applied to phlegm and bile.

There may be a general deficiency of wind together with an extreme deficiency of phlegm and bile; a general deficiency of bile and a great deficiency of phlegm and wind; a general deficiency of phlegm and a great deficiency of wind and bile. Overall, there is a threefold classification of unequal deficiencies among the three humors. For example, there may be a deficiency of wind and bile together with a great deficiency of phlegm; a deficiency of both phlegm and bile with a great deficiency of wind; and a deficiency of both phlegm and wind together with a great deficiency of bile. Those come to a total of twenty-six classes of humoral imbalances.

Among threefold combinations of humoral imbalances, one or two may be in a state of excess while the other one or two are deficient. Wind may generally be in balance while bile is in excess and phlegm is deficient; wind may be in balance, while phlegm is in excess, and bile is deficient. When one adds the same kind of permutation to bile and phlegm, this gives a total of six further classes of humoral imbalances.

Other permutations include deficiencies of both wind and bile together with an excess of phlegm; a deficiency of bile and an excess of both phlegm and wind; a deficiency of phlegm and an excess of both wind and bile; a deficiency of both wind and bile and an excess of phlegm; a deficiency of both phlegm and bile together with an excess of wind; and a deficiency of phlegm and wind together with an excess of bile. Those permutations come to a total of twelve.

In short, there are eighteen types of imbalances of single humors, eighteen types of excess and deficiency of two humors, twenty-six types of excess and deficiency of all three humors, and twelve types of complex imbalances of excess and deficiency, making a total of seventy-four.

There are also cases of "antagonistic" disorders, which begin with an imbalance of one humor, and while it is being treated, another humor becomes imbalanced, but not as a result of improper treatment. For example, while properly treating a wind imbalance, due to the fragility of the patient's constitution, an imbalance of the bile may arise as a side-effect of the medication. The classification of disorders involving detrimental side-effects of medication includes: a bile, phlegm, or bile-and-phlegm imbalance arising before a wind imbalance is cured. The same permutations apply to bile and phlegm, making a total of nine types of disorders.

A related type of disorder entails a kind of "invasion." For example, a common location for wind disorders is in the kidneys and the pelvis. While a wind disorder is present there, a bile or phlegm disorder, or even a threefold combination of wind, bile, and phlegm, may descend upon the kidneys; and that would be an infiltration of a second disorder into the location of the first. Similarly, there may be an invasion of wind into a location of bile, an invasion of phlegm in a location of bile, and an invasion of all three humors into a location of bile; an invasion of wind into a location of phlegm, an invasion of bile into a location of phlegm, and an invasion of all three humors into a location of phlegm. There are nine types of disorders involving such invasions.

To take a specific example, a Tibetan physician may diagnose a disorder as being in the liver or the gall bladder. Most disorders in these two organs entail disorders of the blood, heat, and bile. When detecting a disorder of the liver or gall bladder, many inexperienced Tibetan physicians immediately identify this as a disorder of the blood, heat disorder, or bile. On rare occasions, however, a wind humor may invade the liver or the gall bladder, bringing about a cold wind disorder. If this is not recognized, the physician will prescribe medication that will not only bring no benefit, but will result in abdominal distention and other deleterious side-effects. It is relatively easy to diagnose phlegm disorders, but wind is more difficult, for it is invisible. When trying to identify such a disorder, inexperienced physicians identify a disorder in the liver or the gall bladder and assume (like modern medical doctors) that they are localized in those organs alone. Normally such illnesses occur due to excessive intake of fat, oil, or alcohol, giving rise to a blood disorder and the like. But in the case of a cold wind disorder, that is not always the case. Only decades of experience treating patients enables one to recognize this rare disorder, and only if it is diagnosed properly can one treat it effectively.

I have treated many Western and Asian patients with bile or liver disorders, in which the whites of the eyes, or sclera, become yellow and the skin takes on a yellow tinge. I have found that Tibetan medicine works for all of these people.[36] When the sclera and skin turn yellow, that is called "hepatitis" in the West, but it is not necessarily infectious. But for both the infectious and non-infectious varieties, I have found Tibetan medicine to be generally effective in dispelling such disorders.

To give another example, in the case of chronic headaches, an inexperienced Tibetan physician may automatically assume this involves a bile disorder due to an excessive ingestion of fat or oils, giving rise to a heat disorder. However, in some cases by examining the urine and pulse, one recognizes this as a cold disorder; so all treatment for a bile disorder would be of no benefit.

A final classification of illness pertains to compound, simultaneous imbalances. For example, an imbalance of the life-sustaining wind at the heart may be compounded with an imbalance of phlegm. This is unlike the previous class of illnesses, which were sequential. Further examples of this class of illnesses include: an imbalance of wind in its own location, together with disorders of both phlegm and bile in their own respective locations; and imbalances of bile and phlegm in their own locations, compounded by imbalances of the other humors. Alternatively, a wind imbalance may occur not in its own location but in the location of the bile,

---

36. My translator, Alan Wallace, had hepatitis three times in the early 1970s, and on the third occasion he was close to death. But once he was treated by me, he began to recover overnight.

and it may there come into conflict with phlegm; or a wind imbalance may invade the location of phlegm and then come in conflict with bile.

For example, one of the principal locations of the phlegm is the kidneys. If a wind imbalance invades the kidneys, it may well manifest as a roaring in the ears. An ear specialist may attend solely to the ears, and perhaps prescribe medication for the ears or even surgery, but to no avail. On the other hand, if this patient takes medication to counteract the wind disorder in the kidneys, the symptoms in the ears will vanish. To determine if this is a kidney disorder or some other kind of problem, a Tibetan doctor may question the patient as to the exact type of sound heard in the ears. For example, it could be a high-pitched whine, a swishing sound, or a roaring sound like a jet. These different types of sounds indicate whether the disorder is solely a wind imbalance or a problem of bile or phlegm. Most types of disorders entailing the symptom of sound heard in the ears are due to a wind imbalance. But the wind imbalance may be compounded with an imbalance of bile or phlegm as well. The different types of sounds heard in the ears indicate whether the problem is just a wind disorder or a compound of wind and something else. When such a symptom arises, an ear specialist may do x-rays or probe the ear canal and find nothing at all because there is nothing wrong with the ear. Rather, the origin of the problem is in the kidneys.

Further permutations of this class of disorders pertain to bile: bile may be in a state of imbalance in its own location and come into conflict with both phlegm and wind disorders; bile may invade the location of wind and come into conflict with phlegm; or a bile disorder may invade the location of the phlegm and become compounded with a wind disorder. Likewise, an imbalance of phlegm in its own location may be compounded with imbalances of wind and bile; a phlegm disorder may invade the location of wind and be compounded with a bile disorder; or a phlegm disorder may invade the location of bile and come into conflict with a wind disorder. That makes a total of nine permutations; the preceding three sets of nine make a total of twenty-seven; and the sum total of principal humoral disorders is 101.[37]

---

37. Translator's note: For a somewhat different ordering of this classification of humoral disorders, see the *Encyclopedia of Tibetan Medicine*, Vaidya Bhagwan Dash (Delhi: Sri Satguru Publications, 1994), Vol. II, pp. 160-163. An account similar to, but more concise than, Dr. Dhonden's explanation is found in *The Quintessence Tantras of Tibetan Medicine*, trans. Dr. Barry Clark (Ithaca: Snow Lion, 1995), pp. 91-92.

3. The Classification of Illnesses in Terms of Their Locations

The next class of 101 illnesses is in terms of location, and the two chief locations are the body and mind. The general classifications of disorders in the mind are (1) insanity and (2) amnesia. There are many subclassifications of both, but I shall not go into those. There is a fivefold classification of disorders located in the body: (a) those residing in the upper body, (b) the inner body, (c) the lower body, (d) the outer body, and (e) disorders that pervade the entire body.

(a) Among disorders in the upper body, there are disorders of the (3) head, (4) eyes, (5) ears, (6) nose, (7) lips, (8) teeth, (9) tongue, (10) palate, and (11) goitre. Disorders in the throat include (12) general throat disorders, (13) blockage (e.g., due to tumors in the throat), (14) constriction (due to quinsy, diphtheria, etc.), and (15) speech impediments.

Disorders generally located in the whole head and neck include (16) extreme thirst, (17) hiccups, (18) asthma, of which the Tibetan medical tradition lists seven or eight types, (19) anorxia, and (20) the common cold, of which there are many subclassifications, not all of which are contagious. That makes a total of eighteen types of illnesses of the upper body.

(b) Among disorders of the inner body, there are illnesses of the five solid organs—(21) the heart, (22) lungs, (23) liver, (24) spleen, and (25) kidneys—and the six hollow organs (26) the stomach, (27) gall bladder, (28) small intestine, (29) large intestine, (30) urinary bladder, and (31) the vesicle of regenerative substances. Other illnesses generally located in the solid and hollow organs include (32) indigestion, (33) colic pain due to minute organisms and a conflict between the heat and cold elements of the body,[38] (34) tumors, (35) internal lesions that occur principally in the lungs, liver, kidneys, stomach, large intestine, and spleen, although they may occur in other organs as well,[39] (36) diarrhea due to a heat disorder, and (37) dynsentery.

---

38. To illustrate this, one may first become very cold and then go to a warm place, thereby disturbing the heat and cold elements of the body. This is like pouring boiling water into a glass that was just before filled with ice water. The glass breaks. Such a conflict of heat and cold in the body acts as a catalyst for arousing the activity of small organisms in the body, which act as the direct cause of this disorder.

39. There are eight different types of such internal lesions that appear in the body due to internal causes, particularly impure blood and other types of serous fluids. These lesions are flat (not protruding), round, red, they have a ring around their periphery, and they have a membrane of serous fluid. Because of their red color, round shape, and corona, they are called *sūrya*, which means "sun" in Sanskrit. These

Disorders occurring in the hollow organs alone include (38) diarrhea and (39) vomiting. That makes a total of nineteen types of disorders of the inner body.

(c) Disorders in the lower body, from the waist down, include (40) hemorrhoids, (41) perineal fistula, (42) constipation, (43) anuria, or urinary blockage, and (44) dysuria.

(d) Disorders in the outer body are found in the (i) skin, (ii) flesh, (iii) channels, and (iv) bones.

(*i*) There are ten skin diseases, including: (45) leucoderma, a disease occurring in old and young people alike, which entails dark discoloration of the skin in patches, but with little discomfort; (46) urticaria, which entails redness and flakiness of the skin (as if it has been bruised), but little pain; (47) scabies, or a similar disease entailing dry, itchy skin over the entire body; (48) eczema (or ichthyosis), entailing rough, thick, itchy skin, which becomes stiff like the hide on the back of a bull's neck; (49) a disorder, possibly ringworm, entailing intense itching and small pustules, but no lesions on the skin; (50) blisters that appear all over the skin, from which little pustules form and emit pus[40]; (51) sexually transmitted diseases entailing round lesions initially occurring especially in the mouth and the genitals (if the diseases become chronic, its symptoms spread over the skin); (52) warts; (53) pregnancy mask and other disorders entailing discoloration of the skin around the eyes and ears[41]; (54) and other diseases, including acne, pervading the entire skin.

(*ii*) Disorders of the flesh include (55) goiters, (56) lymphoma, and (57) other diseases that develop in the flesh.

(*iii*) Disorders of the channels include those occurring in the (58) "white channels"—referring to the nervous system—(59) the "dark channels"—which are blood vessels—and (60) other diseases that move through the channels.

---

tend to be chronic, but they can be cured with medication. They are analogous to lesions on the skin where the skin becomes coarse, rippled, tough, thick, and rigid like leather.

40. These pustules range in size from one-half to one inch in diameter, about as big as the tip of a finger, or the biggest would be the tip of the thumb, all over the body. This is not to be confused with contagious skin diseases such as smallpox, chicken pox, and so forth.

41. Although this occurs in both men and women, among women it tends to happen after they have given birth.

(*iv*) Disorders of the bones include (61) gout; (62) elephantiasis, entailing swelling of the legs and discoloration of the skin; (63) other diseases that settle into the bones; and (64) rheumatoid arthritis, which occurs in the flesh, bones, channels, and skin, and entails swelling of the joints, including the fingers, which become crooked, painful and swollen. As far as I know, there is no effective Western medical treatment to cure rheumatoid arthritis, but Tibetan medical treatment can be effective.

(e) Disorders that pervade both the outer and inner regions of the body include (65) diseases of the gall bladder; (66) "brown phlegm" disorders, entailing an imbalance of the wind, bile, phlegm, and blood; (67) ascites; (68) dependent edema[42]; (69) anemia, entailing a pale swelling of the face, limbs, and the rest of the body, as if the blood had drained away[43]; (70) chronic wasting disease, or emaciation; (71) an "unripened" heat disorder,[44] which has not fully developed, (72) a "developing" heat disorder, (73) an "empty" heat disorder, (74) a "hidden" heat disorder, (75) a chronic heat disorder, and (76) a complicated heat disorder[45]; (77) a spreading heat disorder, (78) an agitated heat disorder, (79) a contagious heat disorder; (80) smallpox; (81) hot swelling throughout the body due to a dangerous microorganism; (82) poisoning due to manufactured poisons; (83) air poisoning; (84) poisoning due to the sun's

---

42. In the evening there is swelling in the ankles and the lower legs. If you lie on your right side, the swelling, which is not painful, occurs on the right side of your face and your right leg. If you roll over on your left side, then the swelling occurs on that side. This illness entails an accumulation of water, which moves from one side of the body to another. When you stand up, it accumulates in the lower legs.

43. Unlike dependent edema, this swelling, due to an accumulation of water and serous fluid, remains stationary, without moving around in the body. There are many subclassifications of this disorder involving wind, bile, and phlegm, though most entail imbalances of phlegm and wind. Blood and the bile may be involved, but that is far more rare; and in all cases the pulse is weak and slow.

44. This is a heat disorder that seems to have vanished, like a fire that has been doused with water but is still smoldering. It is called "empty" because its major symptoms have been dispelled due to ingesting cooling medication, but it is still smoldering and is ready to flare up again.

45. These are heat disorders that become complicated by a combining disorder of the serous fluid, which makes for a more serious illness. This is like stirring up the silt on the bottom of a limpid pool of water so that it becomes opaque. The Tibetan names of these six types of heat disorders are: (1) *ma smin*, (2) *rgyas*, (3) *stongs*, (4) *gab*, (5) *rnying*, and (6) *rnyogs*.

rays[46]; (85) poisoning from vapor or airborne moisture coming from the earth; (86) meat poisoning, (87) food poisoning due to unhealthy food combinations; (88) aconite poisoning; (89) rabies; (90) poisoning from scorpions, millipedes, spiders, and insects; (91) poisoning from snakebite; (92) disorders caused by "elemental" demonic forces (*bhūtas*); (93) disorders due to planetary influences; (94) leprosy; (95) a cancerous growth involving chronic, ulcerating lesions on the interior and exterior of the body; (96) erysipelas; (97) parasitic disorders; (98) lesions on the exterior and interior of the head; (99) lesions on the interior and exterior of the torso; (100) lesions on the legs and arms; and (101) lesions on the neck.[47]

This concludes the discussion of the various classifications of diseases.

---

46. In traditional Tibet, when the sun was shining brightly in the morning, people would put blinds on their windows, and they would never think of sun bathing. This type of poisoning can occur during the heat of the day under direct sunlight or even reflected sunlight. Thus, while walking under the midday sun, Tibetans would put something on top of their heads to protect it.

47. Translator's note: Given the time limitations of this lecture series, Dr. Dhonden chose not to discuss the fourth category of 101 disorders according to type, but to proceed to a discussion of medical ethics. In brief, this final class of disorders includes various types of internal diseases, lesions, fevers, and miscellaneous diseases. For a list of these see the *Encyclopedia of Tibetan Medicine*, Vaidya Bhagwan Dash (Delhi: Sri Satguru Publications, 1994), Vol. III, pp. 171-181.

Part III:
Healing from the Source

Chapter Eleven
On Being a Tibetan Physician

In the Tibetan tradition, medical ethics are explained in terms of the following topics: (I) the causes of becoming a physician, (II) the nature of a physician, (III) the designation of a physician, (IV) categories of physicians, (V) the activities of a physician, and (VI) the results of being a physician.

The Causes of Becoming a Physician

Among the six causes of becoming a qualified Tibetan physician are (A) intelligence and understanding, (B) a virtuous motivation, (C) keeping one's pledges, (D) having a thorough knowledge of medicine, (E) dedication to healing, and (F) conduct appropriate to the society in which one is practicing medicine.

(A) The type of intelligence and understanding required on the part of a Tibetan physician is broad-ranging, in the sense of possessing erudition in all the eighteen subcategories of the five fields of knowledge, including the creative arts, medicine, linguistics, logic, and spiritual knowledge.[48] The physician's intelligence should be stable (in the sense of not vacillating) and precise, such that he or she knows how to perform an exact diagnosis and prescribe treatment without hesitation or doubt.

---

48. Translator's note: The eighteen subcategories include: (1) the creative arts, (2) healing, (3) linguistics (specifically Sanskrit grammar), (4) logic, (5) knowledge of the inanimate external universe, (6) knowledge of the characteristics of the six classes of sentient beings who inhabit the universe, (7) knowledge of karma as this pertains

Such precise intelligence also implies having a stable memory, so that one has a clear recollection of all the instructions one has received during one's medical training. Only then can one perform rigorous diagnoses and know the exact types of diet and conduct that the patient should adopt. Thus, precise intelligence must be applied to both diagnosis and treatment.

(B) As for a virtuous motivation, a physician should be imbued with a "spirit of awakening" (*bodhicitta*), which is an altruistic aspiration to achieve spiritual awakening for the benefit of all beings, without discrimination. There are three phases to this spiritual practice: the preparation, the actual practice, and the culmination. The preparation is to cultivate such an altruistic motivation and to take the *bodhisattva* vows[49] that are associated with this spirit of awakening. As a result of this preparation, a physician compassionately looks upon all living beings suffering from illness as if that being were his or her own family member. The actual practice is to engage in the *bodhisattva* way of life, a *bodhisattva*[50] being an individual who is imbued with the motivation of the spirit of awakening and is on the path of awakening.[51] With regard to all sentient

---

to the fortunate and miserable realms of existence, (8) knowledge of the types of rebirth, (9) knowledge of the transitions of birth, dying, and the intermediate state, (10) knowledge of death, (11) knowledge of the different degrees of intelligence, (12) knowledge of the mind by knowing the thoughts of others, (13) knowledge of creation in terms of the five elements, (14) knowledge of the six objects of cognition, (15) knowledge of *mantras* by which all things can be blessed, (16) knowledge of medicine such that the medicinal properties of all things are recognized, (17) knowledge of *dharma*, particularly in terms of the five paths of each of the three spiritual vehicles, and (18) knowledge of spiritual awakening, in which *saṃsāra* and *nirvāṇa* are recognized as being of one nature. [*Chos kyi rnam grangs*, by mGon po dbang rgyal (Chengdu: Sichuan People's Press, 1986), pp. 438-439.]

49. Translator's note: For a description of these vows see Asaṅga & Tsong-Kha-Pa, Asaṅga's Chapter on Ethics with the Commentary of Tsong-Kha-Pa, *The Basic Path to Awakening, The Complete Bodhisattva*, trans. Mark Tatz (Lewiston: Edwin Mellen Press, 1986) (Studies in Asian Thought and Religion), Vol. 4.

50. Translator's note: Tib. *byang chub sems dpa'*. A being in whom the spirit of awakening has effortlessly arisen and who devotes himself or herself to the cultivation of the six perfections in order to achieve spiritual awakening for the benefit of all beings.

51. Translator's note: A definitive presentation of the *bodhisattva* way of life is to be found in Śāntideva, *A Guide to the Bodhisattva Way of Life*, trans. Vesna A. Wallace and B. Alan Wallace (Ithaca: Snow Lion Publications, 1997).

beings in general and one's own patients in particular, the doctor should never consider the financial status of others and or be concerned with his or her own financial remuneration from giving treatment. Regardless of the patients' ability to compensate the physician, the quality of treatment must be the same for all.

The essence of this way of life is to cultivate and embody the "four immeasurables": compassion, loving-kindness, empathetic joy, and impartiality.[52] Compassion in this regard entails being unable to bear the suffering of any sentient being, especially due to illness, and wishing them to be free from suffering. Loving-kindness entails looking upon others with the sense that they are one's own loved ones or relatives, and wishing to bring them happiness. Empathetic joy enables one to treat all patients equally, without regard for their ability to give anything in return. Impartiality is cultivated towards all those who are ill, regardless of their wealth, status, or the ways they have behaved towards one in the past. For example, a physician must treat with impartiality those who have been his worst enemies in the past and those who have been of great benefit to himself or his family.

The physician's motivation is first of all to heal the patient, but he or she also prays that a spirit of awakening may eventually arise in the patients' minds, and that they may proceed on the path to enlightenment. Moreover, the doctor must treat all patients without regard for his own reputation, and he must not be fainthearted in his service to others, anxiously worrying about whether his treatment will be effective. In addition, the doctor must not place conditions on giving treatment. For example, if the patient has cheated the physician in the past, he must never let that influence his present treatment. If the patient is ill, proper treatment must be given without stipulations.

If the physician treats his patients with altruism and follows the conduct of a *bodhisattva*, this enhances his power to heal. This is an invisible factor that influences the efficacy of medical treatment. While it is the medication that directly and overtly benefits the patient, the hidden therapeutic factor empowering the medicine is the altruistic motivation of the doctor. In traditional Tibet, a relative of an invalid might be sent to fetch a doctor on horseback to come and make a house-call. Since trans-

---

52. Translator's note: A detailed explanation of ways to cultivate the four immeasurables is presented in B. Alan Wallace, *Boundless Heart: The Four Immeasurables* (Ithaca: Snow Lion, 1999).

portation was so slow, this might take a couple of days. A horse would be brought to the physician's home, and with great respect he would be asked to accompany the messenger, who would lead him to the home of the patient. In many cases, due to the altruism of the physician, the patient would begin to recover as soon as the doctor arrived, before any medication had been prescribed.

(C) There are six aspects to keeping one's pledges.

(1) The first of these is the cultivation of six attitudes.

(a) The first is the attitude of a physician toward his own teacher. Regardless of whether the teacher is a lay person, a monk, or a *lama,* a doctor should look upon his teacher as if he or she were a *buddha,* or perfectly enlightened being. Since the doctor is not able to encounter the Medicine Buddha himself, he should regard his own teacher as being a *buddha.*

(b) A doctor should have the attitude of regarding the instructions he has received from his teacher as if they had all the authenticity of the instructions of the Buddha himself.

(c) A doctor should have the attitude of regarding medical texts as the words of the Buddha as well as of the *tantras.*

(d) A doctor should have the attitude of regarding his fellow medical practitioners as if they were his own relatives.

(e) His attitude toward patients—whether they are his friends, enemies or complete strangers—should be to compassionately regard them as if they were his own children, speaking gently to them and doing all he can to alleviate their illness.

(f) A doctor should have the attitude of viewing all the disagreeable emissions from patients—including pus, blood, excrement, urine, and so forth—with complete equanimity, feeling no more repugnance than would a dog or a pig.

(2) The second pledge for a Tibetan doctor is to properly maintain two things, the first of which is regarding each holder of medical knowledge as a protector of the words of the Buddha; and the second is regarding medical instruments as the various items held by such a protector.

(3) Third among the pledges are "three things to be known," which are actually three attitudes regarding one's medication: to look upon them as precious substances, as ambrosia, and as offerings. In the medical colleges

of traditional Tibet, medical ingredients would be gathered, and at a certain point in the year these would all be compounded into medicines and then laid out in a large *maṇḍala,* or symbolic diagram. In the *maṇḍala* they are empowered with rituals, meditation, and devotions, and they were then offered to the *buddhas* and *bodhisattvas.* This was a way of making an offering to these objects of refuge and also of blessing those medications.

When the Chinese invaded and occupied Tibet, they regarded all religion as poison, and though they encouraged Tibetan medicine and allowed medications to be made, they secularized it in the process. For example, they prohibited Tibetans from engaging in any spiritual practices regarding the production and distribution of their medication. Throughout the Cultural Revolution, it was illegal to lay the medicines on a *maṇḍala,* but by the end of the 1970s, Chinese authorities had noted that Tibetan medications were not as effective as they had been before these prohibitions. So they changed the rules back and allowed the Tibetan doctors to prepare and bless the medicines as they had done previously, which restored the efficacy of these medications. For example, a class of medicines known as "precious pills" are now being made in large quantities in Tibet, and the Chinese are retailing them through Hong Kong, for they have found them to be very effective

Medications are to be looked upon as wish-fulfilling jewels because they provide a physician with all his needs for making a living; and they are looked upon as if they were ambrosia because they swiftly eliminate illnesses, thus enabling patients to "cheat death." Since the medicines are immediately offered to the enlightened beings as soon as they are prepared, they are regarded as offerings.

Just as a miner seeks out jewels, so does a physician seek medicinal substances at the appropriate time and place and in the correct manner. For example, a physician must know the seasons in which specific medicinal plants are to be gathered, as well as the manner and place in which they are to be collected. There are also proper ways to collect medicinal mineral substances.

Once a medicine has been prepared, as I mentioned previously, it is set out on a *maṇḍala* as part of the ritual offering; and then the physician engages in the two stages of tantric meditation known as the *stage of generation* and the *stage of completion*.[53] Afterwards, the physician utters auspicious verses to bring forth the greatest possible benefit from the medication and then recites *mantras* to enhance the efficacy of the medicines. The next phase of this ritual is to offer the medicines to the *vidyādharas*,[54] or "holders of pristine awareness," which is an epithet of the *buddhas*. Specifically, one offers the medicines to the entire lineage of teachers of medicine, going back to the Medicine Buddha and to Buddha Śākyamuni. In so doing, one makes offerings to Buddhist and non-Buddhist deities, teachers, and physicians, for no discrimination is to be made between Buddhists and non-Buddhists. After making these offerings, the doctor ingests a small, symbolic amount of the medication himself, so that he receives the blessing of these medications that have been so empowered.

(D) Having a thorough knowledge of medicine pertains to the role of the doctor's body, speech, and mind in the preparation and dispensing of medicines. With his body, a physician makes and dispenses medical compounds and gives other types of medical treatment, such as moxibustion, taking blood and so forth. With his speech, a physician should address his patients with gentle words of encouragement as if they were his own loved ones and relatives. He should never speak harshly or out of irritation, but should do all he can to comfort and encourage his patients. With his mind, a physician should clearly recollect the knowledge he has acquired and know exactly how to apply this in pulse diagnosis and urine analysis. He should have a clear sense of the type of medication that will be of benefit and, where appropriate, the proper sequence of medicines to be administered. He should be able to treat his patients as if he were clairvoyant.

(E) Dedication to healing is a way of fulfilling one's own needs and the welfare of others. The point is that if one does not attend to one's own need to become a good physician, one cannot serve the interests of others. In terms of one's own needs, a student must cultivate the causes

---

53. Translator's note: Explanations of these two phases of tantric practice, specifically for Kālacakra practice, are found in Gen Lamrimpa, *Transcending Time: An Explanation of the Kālacakra Six-Session Guruyoga*, trans. B. Alan Wallace (Boston: Wisdom, 1999).

54. Translator's note: Tib. *rig pa 'dzin pa*. A "holder of knowledge," who has ascertained the nature of pristine awareness.

of becoming a qualified physician by first thoroughly studying all the great medical treatises. Having learned them completely, one debates their subtle points and learns how to compose one's own treatises or commentaries on the classics. Such training is the primary cause of becoming a physician, and a contributing circumstance is devoting oneself to a fully qualified teacher.

A fully qualified physician should have a thorough knowledge of Buddhist and non-Buddhist medical treatises. Such vast erudition provides one with an all-encompassing view like that of a person who has climbed to the top of a mountain peak and can see a vast panorama in all directions. A doctor should have a serene demeanor, few material desires, be able to explain things clearly, have integrity, and a merciful attitude towards his patients and students. Once one finds such a teacher who is a fully qualified physician, one should single-pointedly entrust oneself to this person's guidance and follow him or her without hypocrisy; that is, with one's inner attitude being congruent with one's outer behavior. As one devotes oneself to such a teacher, one should always gratefully bear in mind his great kindness. If one relates to a qualified teacher in the proper manner, one will swiftly gain mastery of this discipline.

In addition, one should be conscientious with regards to the kind of company one keeps. If one accompanies people who are lazy and idle away their time, such companionship will be an obstacle to completing one's medical training. One's companions should be exemplary students who are devoted to their studies. By devoting oneself to such colleagues, one's own needs are more easily fulfilled. As for fulfilling others' needs, one should avoid procrastination in treating patients. Moreover, one must be meticulous in performing pulse diagnosis and urine analysis for the patient. To illustrate the degree of care one should take, imagine that you must walk with a pot full of oil on your head over a plank that has been laid from the roof of one tall building to another. If just one drop spills from the pot, you will be executed on the spot. The physician should be just as meticulous when diagnosing the pulse and urine, maintaining single-pointed concentration all the while.

(F) Conduct appropriate to the society in which one is practicing medicine has to do with both worldly and religious customs. This is to say that one should act in accordance with the worldly religious norms of the people one is treating. In short, one should always behave with modesty and humility toward everyone, regardless of their degree of affluence or social status. According to the Tibetan custom, one should show great deference toward one's father and mother, toward the elderly, toward monks and lamas, and also toward people in the government.

The Nature of a Physician

A qualified Tibetan physician must thoroughly fathom all aspects of the body, including the ten afflicted elements of the body and the fifteen subclassifications of the three humors, both in their balanced and imbalanced states. He should also be well versed in all types of conduct, diet, and medical treatment prescribed as remedies for treating the individual when there is a condition of imbalance.

The Designation of a Physician

The Tibetan word for physician (*sman pa*) has the same connotation as the Tibetan verb "to benefit" (*phan pa*). Thus, a physician is said to be one who benefits others by curing illnesses.

Categories of Physicians

There are three types of physicians: unsurpassed, expert, and ordinary. The category of "unsurpassed physician" refers to the Medicine Buddha alone, because he is the Supreme Physician who dispels the afflictions of the three poisons of attachment, hatred, and delusion, together with their consequences. An expert physician is one who possesses clairvoyance, who knows the minds of others, and is imbued with loving-kindness and integrity. Such a doctor is able to discern every type of illness by means of his extrasensory perception,[55] without having to rely upon the patient's account of the illness. Then with a motivation of compassion and loving-kindness, he is able to pacify all manner of illnesses, like a *buddha* who has pacified his own afflictions and thereby is able to pacify the afflictions of others.

An ordinary physician is one who becomes a doctor with the self-centered aspiration to make a living, and to acquire reputation and wealth.

---

55. Translator's note: For an explanation of ways to cultivate extrasensory perception using Buddhist techniques for enhancing the attention, see B. Alan Wallace, *The Bridge of Quiescence: Experiencing Tibetan Buddhist Meditation* (Chicago: Open Court, 1998).

Someone who enters the medical profession with such a motivation is said to be in the same class as a butcher. Ordinary physicians achieve their position in various ways: (1) some receive their license from a governmental agency or are authorized to practice by their own private teacher, for whom they have served as an apprentice; (2) some simply mimic the practice of qualified doctors, but even they may be of some benefit; (3) some, out of a desire for reputation, acquire medical instruments and simply pretend to practice medicine, even though they have no knowledge of medicine; (4) some practice medicine after being chronically ill, healing themselves, and applying their limited knowledge to others; (5) some are dilettantes who have learned a few medical phrases and a few medications, then take on the role of a physician; (6) some are impostors who have not studied under any teacher but have acquired notes or prescriptions of others and then claim to be doctors themselves; and (7) some are pharmacists who learn of medicines that are helpful for specific illnesses, go into the business selling those medicines, and on that basis call themselves doctors.

If a Tibetan doctor practices medicine unrelated to any spiritual practice, this can act as a cause of suffering. This runs against the grain of the modern world, in which the medical profession and pharmaceutical companies are so attentive to making profit. This is antithetical to the spirit of Tibetan medicine, even though there may be some immediate, short-term benefit for patients. Karmically speaking, the long-term consequences of practicing medicine with a self-centered motivation are an unfortunate rebirth and suffering for oneself. Therefore, it is very important to integrate one's spiritual practice with one's medical practice so that they work together to alleviate suffering.

In order to engage in spiritual practice, one should find a qualified spiritual mentor, and not just follow after any charismatic teacher. Thus, one should carefully examine a spiritual mentor before accepting him or her as one's own guide. Once one has ascertained that a teacher is indeed qualified to guide one on the path to enlightenment, one should attend well, for such a person will not lead one astray. In Tibet for example, there were people who called themselves *lamas* without having any qualifications at all. Not all qualified spiritual teachers were monks; in fact, there have been many superb lay teachers in the history of Tibetan Buddhism, such as Marpa, the great translator who was the *lama* of Milarepa, perhaps the most renowned of all Tibetan contemplatives.

In terms of the genealogy of the healer, there were physicians of different social classes both in India and Tibet, including the noble class (*kṣatriya*), the priestly class (*brahmin*), the class of the general populace (*vaiśya*), and the lowest class of society (*vṛṣala*). On the whole, physicians would be drawn from any of the upper three classes, but not the lowest. Generally speaking, the whole of Buddhism, from the basic monastic discipline up to the esoteric teachings of the Vajrayāna, is egalitarian in the sense of showing no preference for any social class.

The first characteristic of an excellent healer is that he or she is born of a noble lineage, stemming from great Buddhist teachers, such as the lineage of Marpa, his disciple Ngok Chöku Dorje, the Khön lineage of the Sakya order, and the family line of Thönmi Sambhoṭa, who devised the Tibetan alphabet and grammar. In Tibet family lines are both patrilineal and matrilineal.

In my own lineage it was the custom for all the sons to become either *lamas* or monks. To become a *lama*, or spiritual master, one does not necessarily have to become a monk, which entails taking monastic precepts including chastity. If a father in my lineage had three sons, the first son, according to tradition, would become a *lama*, but one who could and should take a wife and have children. The other sons would become monks, who would remain celibate. The principal responsibility of the first son was to become a tantric adept who could control the weather, especially averting hail storms. However, if the eldest son failed to produce a male heir, then a divination would be performed to choose one of the other sons to return from the monastery, become a *lama*, and raise a family.

My lineage traces back to Ngok Chöku Dorje, an erudite Nyingma *lama* of the twelfth century who eventually trained under the great Kagyü master Marpa. To show his utter dedication and commitment to the Dharma and his *lama*, Ngok Chöku Dorje offered all his worldly goods— including his sheep, yaks, dogs, and everything else—to Marpa in order to receive teachings. He lived about four or five days' journey from Marpa, and when he rounded up all his livestock as an offering, he excluded one lame goat that he thought was unfit for the journey. When he presented all this wealth to his *lama*, Marpa replied, "What about that lame goat? You said you were offering me everything. I want the lame goat too!" So he hiked back and brought the lame goat on his shoulders to Marpa, who then accepted him as a disciple. Then Marpa prophesied, "As a karmic consequence of your great devotion, for generations to come, your lineage will always prosper for as long as the Buddhadharma remains." From that point, Ngok Chöku Dorje became a *lama* of the Kagyü order.

The other qualifications of an excellent Tibetan doctor are intelligence, maintaining one's tantric pledges, erudition, the ability to synthesize one's textual knowledge in actual practice, strong devotion to spiritual practice, freedom from sensual craving, a subdued and disciplined demeanor, skill in making medicines, and great loving-kindness for all living beings. A doctor should have an unwavering attitude of attending to the needs of others as if they were his own needs, and he should have no confusion with regard to all types of medical treatment. Those are the qualifications of an excellent doctor, and such a person is said to be the sole protector of all living beings who are ill. This person should be "a child of the lineage," in the sense of preserving the lineage of the medical teachings tracing back to the Buddha. A doctor who is endowed with all the previous characteristics is said to be a veritable emanation of the Medicine Buddha.

There is another list of characteristics of a person who has inadequate qualifications to serve as a doctor. Although a qualified doctor may be a commoner who does not belong either to a noble lineage or a lineage of doctors who treated royalty, (1) it is improper for a person with a despised family background to become a physician. The reason is that the society will not respect such a person or honor him as a doctor, so his ability to serve in the role of a healer would be impaired. In short, apart from the class of people who make their living by killing, a physician can be of any class.

A second quality of incompetence as a doctor is (2) lack of knowledge of the medical treatises. Like someone wandering in the dark, such a person does not know how to diagnose or treat patients, so he cannot be effective in his role as a doctor. A doctor is inadequate (3 & 4) if he has not observed a skilled physician in practice and gained sustained experience, or familiarity, as an apprentice. A true apprentice will learn through experience by watching a master physician in action, seeing how the urine is analyzed and the pulse is diagnosed. Like someone who sets out on a road without knowing where he is going, a person without such experience as an apprentice becomes filled with uncertainty when trying to diagnose and treat illnesses.

(5) Ignorance of the correct methods of diagnosing the pulse and urine is another sign of incompetence, for such a person will not be able to "hear the voices" of illnesses as they are expressed in the pulse and urine.

(6) Ignorance of how to read an astrological ephemeris and make correct inferences pertaining to medical treatment is another liability for a doctor, for this will impair the efficacy of his treatment.

Although one may know how to diagnose illnesses, (7) if one does not know how to treat illnesses correctly, one is incompetent. Like shooting an arrow at a target in the dark, the prescribed antidotes will not correspond to the illnesses in need of cure.

Although a physician may be able to prescribe proper treatment, if (8) he does not know how to prescribe the correct diet and conduct, he is incompetent, for unhealthy diet and conduct is bound to undermine the efficacy of the medication.

If a patient has a heat disorder, a Tibetan physician will prescribe cooling medication, cooling food, and behavior to alleviate that illness. Then as the heat disorder gradually subsides, the medication should correspondingly be altered over time. (9) A healer who does not know how to give medical treatments appropriate to calming such disturbances is like a farmer who does not know how to tend his field. Such a person is prone to exacerbating illnesses due to improper treatment.

(10) For some illnesses a laxative is prescribed, and for others an emetic is needed. If a physician prescribes one of these treatments when the other is needed, he is incompetent. When this happens, an illness may be flushed from the system together with elements of the seven bodily constituents, resulting in a loss of vitality. This is like pouring water on a mound of sand, such that the sand and the water both flow away.

(11) A doctor without medical instruments is incompetent, like a warrior who ventures into battle with no weapons.

(12) A doctor who does not know how to perform moxibustion, bloodletting, or surgery is incompetent. For example, a doctor may be confused as to whether fluid should be drawn from the right or the left lung; or if surgery is needed, he may not know which organ to operate on. Such a doctor is like a thief who hears of a wealthy household that he wants to rob, but instead of locating that house, he breaks into another one that is empty.

A doctor who is incompetent in any of the above ways is to be avoided, for he is like someone who wields the instruments of the Lord of Death.

The Activities of a Physician

There are both common and special activities of a Tibetan physician. Common bodily activities include gathering medicinal herbs, preparing medical compounds, using instruments such as in moxibustion, and performing pulse diagnosis and urinalysis. In terms of the common activities of the speech, a doctor should be able to point out the nature and origins of the illness to the patient, and explain how it is to be treated, including the behavior and diet to be followed by the patient. Moreover, a physician should be able to state whether or not the patient will survive the illness. However, even if a physician sees that the condition is a fatal one, he may not tell the patient that he will die, but will instead encourage the patient to engage in spiritual practices such as prayer and taking refuge. On the other hand, a physician may tell the relatives of the patient that they should prepare for his death. Actually, on most occasions in Tibet dying patients themselves, especially experienced religious practitioners, knew they were going to die, either on the basis of their symptoms or premonitions in dreams. In those cases it would be the patient who told the physician that he was going to die.

The Cultural Revolution in the 1960s and '70s was the darkest hour in the history of Tibet, when Tibetan culture and religion were most fiercely attacked by the Chinese Communists. During that period, it was against the law to practice religion in Tibet, but even then some people continued to meditate. Some who were incarcerated in concentration camps died and in so doing displayed extraordinary degrees of spiritual realization, including the achievement of the "rainbow body." I have met a number of people who have left Tibet since then who have witnessed this for themselves. In one case, a Tibetan contemplative who was a very large man died, and his body then shrank down to the size of about one cubit. This indicates an exceptionally high degree of spiritual maturation, even though that is not the actual rainbow body. One who has fully achieved the rainbow body at death completely dissolves the body into space like a rainbow in the sky, leaving only the hair and nails behind. This has not occurred recently, but there have been many cases of the corpse of a contemplative shrinking dramatically right after death. This has been witnessed by many people.

When I was a young boy of eight or nine years, before I went to Lhasa to study medicine, I lived in Sungrab Ling Monastery in which lived an old monk named Döndrub. Every morning Döndrub was in the habit of preparing little balls of parched barley meal as ritual offerings to the *buddhas*, the Dharma protectors, and all sentient beings. This ritual would take about a half hour. To me, his spiritual practice seemed to be very simple. He would pray to Tārā, the feminine embodiment of enlightened compassion, and to Avalokiteśvara, the masculine embodiment of compassion.

One evening it was cold and the monks were sitting around a fire on which they were cooking some soup, and this old monk, Döndrub, was joking around with me and commented, "Tomorrow I won't be going to the prayer assembly." I asked, "Why not?" And he replied, "This is none of your business, but don't expect me at prayers tomorrow." I then said, "In that case, I'll make you tea," since he would otherwise miss his morning tea, which was served during the prayer assembly. Actually, Döndrub did not normally go to the prayer assembly anyway, but remained in his room, which was adjacent to mine, engaging in his own spiritual practice. While he was practicing in solitude in his room, the sun would shine through the window in the morning, and he would place a cloth on his head to protect himself from the sun while he performed his devotions. The next morning I brought him his tea, and he said, "Bring me some cheese and *tsampa* (parched barley meal) as well." I did so, and as soon as he finished eating, he carefully cleaned out his bowl, wrapped it up, and told me to put it away. Normally, he would not take such care in cleaning his bowl, but in this case, he was very meticulous. Döndrub then asked me what time it was. I replied, "The prayer assembly is almost over," which was about mid-morning. He commented, "Oh, it's getting a bit too late." I thought that was a funny thing for him to say as he was just sitting there while I was waiting around thinking that the tea was getting cold and going to waste. So I waited to see what he was going to do next. Then he simply slumped over. I went over to him to see if he had fallen asleep, only to discover he had passed away.

I then became quite scared and wondered what had I done. Had I inadvertently poisoned his tea? Would the other monks blame me? At that time in the morning, there were about three hundred monks circumambulating the monastery and I called one of them to see what had happened. This monk was also quite surprised, but when I told him how Döndrub had been acting so unusually that morning, he said that was an indication that the old monk had a degree of spiritual realization. He reassured me it was not my fault and said he would tell the authorities in the monastery what had happened. The elders of the monastery came and ascertained that he was dead, and they all pulled their upper robes around their shoulders and bowed to him to show their final respects. It was at that moment that I knew for sure that Döndrub had died. That was my first encounter in this lifetime with death.

My second experience with death also occurred in Sungrab Ling Monastery a year or so later. At that time, there was an old physician-monk named Khyenrab Ösel who had trained in the Chakpori medical college in Lhasa, founded during the reign of the Fifth Dalai Lama (1617-1682).[56] When he became quite old, he returned to Sungrab Ling. Although he had a number of relatives who lived in that region, they were very busy, so I volunteered to take care of him as if I were his servant. For example, he was quite feeble, so I would help him walk to the urinal. Khyenrab Ösel always encouraged me to study medicine rather than engage in Buddhist scholastic studies. He thought the latter, which involved a lengthy training in debate and dialectics, simply made people arrogant, whereas by studying medicine I could be of practical benefit to others.

In the seventh lunar month (around September), when the monks' summer retreat was over, it was traditional for the monks to go picnicking for a few days. Khyenrab Ösel asked me, "Do you want to join the other monks on the picnic?" I replied, "No, I think I'll stay here." Then he asked what the lunar date was, and I told him it was about the sixth day of the month. He thought I was mistaken, so we fetched a calendar and saw it was the eighth day of the month. That afternoon I stayed with him and brought him some tea. He once again encouraged me to cultivate compassion and study medicine, rather than philosophy, because this is a good way to serve others; and he told me he would pray for me. Then he said, "Now I am going to my room, and I don't want you to come there until everyone else returns from the picnic." I asked him why, and he simply replied, "Just do as I say."

I remained in the monastery for awhile, but the only monks there were the caretakers who guarded the monastery from thieves. On the

---

56. The monastery in Tibet where Dr. Dhonden eventually practiced medicine after his formal training was called Shädrub Ling (bShad sgrub gling), which was also founded during the reign of the Fifth Dalai Lama.

tenth day of the month,[57] after two days of waiting by myself, I became bored, so I joined the others at the picnic. Some of them, including the relatives of Khyenrab Ösel, asked why I had come, for they thought I was going to stay at the monastery. I felt uncomfortable at this point, for I thought I might have upset them in some way. I told them that Khyenrab Ösel told me not to come to his room until everyone had returned from the picnic on the tenth day of the month. At this point they took my words very seriously, and their expressions all changed. Late in the afternoon they all returned from the picnic (normally, they would not return until the evening), and the old monk's relatives went to his room, where they found him sitting slumped over in a meditative posture. As his final act, he had set out offerings to the *buddhas,* then sat in meditation and died. That was my second encounter with death.

I narrate both these accounts to indicate that there were many cases in Tibet, even in my own lifetime, of spiritual adepts knowing with certainty when they would die, preparing for the event, then dying with full consciousness. I have witnessed such events with my own eyes, and if one looks further back in the history of Tibet, there are more extraordinary, authentic accounts of adepts achieving the rainbow body.[58]

To return to the topic at hand, with respect to the special activities of a Tibetan doctor, he should dedicate himself to an authentic view of reality, meditation, and appropriate conduct. In terms of the view, a physician should realize the Madhyamaka (Middle Way) view of the nature of both conventional and ultimate truth, which avoids philosophical extremes. Likewise, in terms of his medical practice, he should also have the Middle View free of the extremes of giving too little medication, too

---

57. This day of the lunar month is considered to be an auspicious, holy day among Tibetan Buddhists.

58. Translator's note: The following is a more recent account of the death of a Tibetan lama, which also illustrates the way in which death itself can be transformed into spiritual practice. On March 31, 1998, in Ka-Nying Shedrub Ling Monastery in Boudhanath, Nepal, the Chant Leader, Lama Putse, died of a chronic respiratory ailment, and he remained for eleven days in what Tibetans believe to be a post-death meditative state. During that time, observers reported, there were none of the usual signs of decay after death. His body remained fresh and completely odor-free, the flesh soft and supple with no sign of rigor mortis. His face was composed and lifelike. On the evening of April 8, Dr. David R. Shlim, a respected chief physician of CIWEC Clinic, came to the monastery to view Lama Putse. Dr. Shlim was astonished at the extraordinary condition of the body and remarked that he

much medication, or the wrong medication. In terms of meditation, a doctor should cultivate the four immeasurables of loving-kindness, compassion, empathetic joy, and impartiality. In terms of behavior, a physician should maintain ethical conduct, specifically by avoiding nonvirtues and all other improper conduct due to intoxication and other mind-altering substances. In terms of medical treatment, a physician should have precise knowledge, with no guesswork, of what should be done for the patient.

There are certain types of conduct to be followed and other types of conduct to be avoided. Among the conduct to be avoided, one should first of all avoid taking the life of anyone, human or non-human, adults or infants. Other physical nonvirtues to avoid are stealing and cheating others out of their wealth, and engaging in sexual misconduct. Nonvirtues having to do with the speech include lying, slander, idle gossip, and abuse. The principal nonvirtues of the mind are avarice, malice, and holding false views. Those are the most important nonvirtues to be avoided.

In terms of the conduct to be followed, a physician should dedicate himself to the perfection of generosity such that he is willing to make any sacrifice necessary for the sake of his patients. He should cultivate the perfection of ethical discipline by doing whatever is needed for his patients, without deviousness, hypocrisy, or expectation of reward. He should cultivate the perfection of patience, especially with respect to all the annoyances, abuse, and complaints he may receive from patients and medical assistants. In addition, he should cultivate the perfection of zeal, completely free of spiritual sloth, such that he is delighted to do whatever is needed for the sake of the ill.

---

could think of no explanation, from either a medical or scientific standpoint, for such an occurrence. On April 9, Dr. Prativa Pandey, also a senior physician of CIWEC Clinic, examined the body and declared that after death, Lama Putse appeared to be demonstrating very rare supramundane qualities that defied scientific explanation. During these eleven days, the room in which his body was laid to rest had a very mild pleasant fragrance and a noticeable freshness. On April 11, the post-death meditation apparently came to an end, and the body began to decompose rapidly. At this point, according to Tibetan Buddhist belief, the subtle consciousness of the contemplative deliberately separates from the physical body.

For an explanation of practices to be performed at the time of death according to the Tibetan Buddhist tradition, see *Natural Liberation: Padmasambhava's Teachings on the Six Bardos*, comm. by Gyatrul Rinpoche; trans. by B. Alan Wallace (Boston: Wisdom Publications, 1998), Ch. 6.

The above four qualities of generosity, ethical discipline, patience, and zeal are the first four of the six perfections that form the framework of the *bodhisattva* way of life. The final two are meditation and wisdom, which I discussed previously in my comments on the view, meditation, and conduct. A doctor's meditation should focus on the cultivation of the four immeasurables, and his cultivation of wisdom should focus on realizing the view of the Middle Way.

The Results of Being a Physician

There are both temporal and ultimate results of being a physician. A temporal result is a great deal of satisfaction in this life. As a result of a physician's cultivation of the four immeasurables and other virtues such as altruism and generosity, one ascends to a position of influence and prosperity. The source of these benefits is medicine itself, which is a reason why one should study well. In terms of the ultimate benefits of being a physician, those who dedicate themselves to healing the ill, without deviousness, hypocrisy, or sensual craving, ultimately attain the state of perfect spiritual awakening. The Medicine Buddha himself has said this is the ultimate result of being a physician who follows such conduct, regardless of one's race or religion.

Chapter Twelve
A Tibetan Medical View of AIDS

From a Tibetan medical perspective, the disease presently known as AIDS is included in a category of eighteen microbial and infectious diseases. This category also includes the various forms of cancer. The eighteen microbial and infectious diseases are all explained in *The Oral Instruction Tantra*, taught by Ratnasambhava, and a clear commentary on this class of diseases is found in Sangye Gyatso's *Supplement to The Oral Instruction Tantra*

In beginning of *The Oral Instruction Tantra*, Ratnasambhava declares that among the six classes of sentient beings, humans are foremost in terms of our intelligence and powers of discernment; but due to ignorance, we continue to revolve in the cycle of existence known as *saṃsāra*.[59] Among the other classes of sentient beings, *devas* (gods) are impaired by their infatuation with sensual pleasures. *Asuras* (demigods) are impaired by their jealousy and aggression. Animals, on the whole, are impaired by the dullness of their intelligence. *Pretas* (spirits) are impaired by their intense craving and powerful, unsatiated hunger and thirst. Finally, the denizens of various finite, but terribly painful, hell realms are impaired by intense sufferings of heat or cold and so forth. In comparison with these other classes of sentient beings, human beings have the greatest potentiality especially due to our intelligence.

---

59. Translator's note: *Saṃsāra* is the cycle of existence, qualified by compulsively taking rebirth after rebirth due to the power of one's mental afflictions and *karma*.

Five mental poisons have principal roles in perpetuating our existence in the cycle of *saṃsāra*. The most fundamental of these are ignorance and delusion, specifically in terms of failing to distinguish between wholesome and unwholesome conduct. Secondly, most vices stem from attachment and craving, which motivate us to acquire material possessions and so forth, which, in turn, often leads to such actions as killing, lying, and so on. The third mental poison, hatred, causes us to inflict harm upon others, both physically and verbally. The fourth poison of jealousy engenders an attitude of competitiveness toward our superiors. When countries are dominated by jealousy, they compete with one another, each one trying to outdo its neighbors in the development of more powerful weapons and technology. The fifth poison of pride entails a sense of one's own superiority and a dismissive attitude toward others.

Even though human beings are exceptionally intelligent in the overall scheme of things, our intelligence is all too often applied solely to the acquisition of material prosperity and so forth, without taking into account future lives and the long-term consequences of our deeds. In this way, intelligence itself tends to stimulate the five poisons, which create imbalances in the three humors. Therefore, it is said that due to the influence of mental afflictions on the three humors, all the 404 classifications of illnesses arise in an unbroken stream, such that there is never a time when one is completely at ease or completely happy.

Following *The Oral Instruction Tantra, The Final Tantra* was revealed by Amoghasiddhi. Upon its conclusion, Manasija, who had requested this *tantra,* asked about the nature, diagnosis, and treatment of illnesses that would arise during the final five hundred years of the duration of the Buddha's teachings, when society is dominated by the five types of degeneration. This last period of five hundred years began, I believe, in the eighteenth century, and it is an era in which it is prophesied that vices and material affluence will increase, while virtue will decline. This is a period in which promises, oaths, and vows will be broken in personal, governmental, and business affairs. False views will proliferate. People will reject or ignore the truth of the continuity of consciousness from one life to the next, while assuming that death entails total, personal annihilation. People will reject the possibility of effective practices that result in spiritual maturation. Moreover, people of all religious faiths, including Buddhism, will give only lip service to their objects of refuge. Even monks and nuns will hold false views, fail to keep their precepts, and take monastic vows only as a means to gain a livelihood and acquire social status, reputation, respect from others, and so forth. This is an era in which so-called religious people will not actually practice their religions, but rather treat them as merchandise, to be sold at profit.

Engaging in the esoteric practices of Vajrayāna Buddhism can lead to swift spiritual realization, at which point one is qualified to give tantric initiations, oral transmissions, and teachings. However, people in this degenerate era who engage in such practice, but without carrying through to the point of gaining genuine insight, will still take on the role of being *lamas* and give initiations, even though they are totally unqualified. In this phase of human history, many kings, presidents, prime ministers, and other government officials, as well as the populace as a whole, will lack integrity. Judges and peace officers will turn to bribes, so that governments will be run simply by those who have the most money.

This long prophesy of the present era of degeneration points to the causes and conditions that lead to the above eighteen types of diseases. The *tantra* also states that in this degenerate era, extremists (those who do not embrace any type of spiritual world view or practice, but rather promote materialism and nihilism) will introduce various types of toxic substances into the environment. I surmise that these include the airborne pollutants created by atomic and hydrogen weapons, pesticides, and all types of poisons and contaminants that have been produced by modern industry. According to the Buddhist world view, various types of non-human beings inhabit the sky, and when these poisons become airborne, they poison these beings, making them ill, and the diseases that they experience return into the atmosphere. In this way, unprecedented types of minute organisms are produced in the atmosphere, and they then fall to earth, and these are the immediate causes of these eighteen types of diseases. Thus, these new diseases arise due to a confluence of two influences: the general, moral degeneration of modern society and the production of toxins that enter the atmosphere, which produce new types of harmful organisms that return to earth and spread disease.

According to the *tantra*, these minute organisms have heads like that of a lizard with a big mouth, long tails like that of a snake, and many limbs like those of a centipede. I believe they should be visible through a microscope. They move about freely in the atmosphere, and they can enter the human body by way of the nostrils and through the pores. In addition, the Tibetan medical tradition states there are seven types of minute organisms that are native to the human body,[60] the smallest of which is invisible to the naked eye, even though they should be visible through a microscope. These tiniest organisms are red in color, they circulate rapidly through the body in the bloodstream, and they by themselves are not detrimental to one's health. However, when the above-mentioned airborne organisms come into contact with the minute, red organisms in the bloodstream, disorders involving the three humors arise due to the conjoining of these two types of organisms.

All the eighteen disorders of this category (*gnyan rims*) originate in this fashion. Among those eighteen is one subclass of diseases (*gnyan*) that originate from minute organisms, but which are not infectious.[61] The various kinds of cancer generally belong to that category. The second subclass (*rims*) consists of infectious diseases that can be transmitted by one contaminated person breathing or coughing on another, although the easiest way to transmit such diseases is through blood transfusions.

As the harmful organisms that were originally airborne course through the body, they do so in dependence upon the four elements. They are like a horseman who rides the mount of the four elements. Recall that phlegm is associated with earth and water, wind with air, and bile with fire. There are three types of disorders of this sort: heat disorders, contagious disorders, and disorders due to minute organisms. All of these entail some kind of heat disorder. Disorders due to minute organisms tend to be the most virulent, for they swiftly turn into serious illnesses. Even though they entail a heat disorder, treatment for heat disorders alone, which cool the body and may suppress the symptoms of the heat disorder itself, will not be effective in eliminating the underlying cause of the illness, which is the organisms. On the other hand, if one gives medication

---

60. More broadly speaking, according to the Buddha, there are 21,000 types of microorganisms within the body, corresponding to 84,000 types of mental afflictions. For each mental affliction there must be a corresponding microorganism, for there is a physiological basis for all mental afflictions. Buddhist scholars study the 84,000 collections of the Buddha's teachings, which are designed to counteract those 84,000 mental afflictions, which are all derivative of the three mental poisons: attachment, hatred, and delusion.

61. Translator's note: The term *gnyan* normally refers to a type of earth spirit (Tib. *sa bdag*, Skt. *kṣamāpati*) that may cause illnesses, but Dr. Dhonden interprets this word as referring to microbes.

designed solely to eliminate those organisms, that alone does not relieve the heat disorder. As an analogy, water can slake one's thirst, but it does not satisfy one's hunger; and solid food can satisfy one's hunger, but it does not alleviate one's thirst. In Western medicine very powerful drugs have been created to kill various types of viruses and bacteria,[62] but since the nature and functioning of the three humors is not generally recognized in the West, simply killing those minute organisms is like either satisfying the hunger or the thirst, but not both. According to Tibetan medicine, it is generally not sufficient to kill the microorganism alone, with no ancillary treatment to balance and restore the body as a whole.

To effectively treat these microbial diseases, one must give different medications for each aspect of the disease, and in some cases the medications must be given sequentially. Moreover, one critical factor for the perpetuation and growth of such diseases is the wind humor, which moves these diseases around the body, causing them to proliferate. The wind humor cannot be detected by modern technology, so the Western medical tradition does not acknowledge its existence. Thus, Western physicians often prescribe localized treatment for various types of tumors including breast cancer. For example, they may detect a tumor in the breast and decide that the breast must be removed, without identifying the underlying cause for the appearance of the cancer itself. The wind humor moves those underlying causes of the specific manifestations of diseases, such as cancer, elsewhere in the body. Therefore, it is ineffective simply to remove the superficial expression of a disease in one area, without eradicating its underlying cause or that which spreads that cause. Consider this carefully. What is it that carries the disease from one place in the body to another? If this is not the wind humor (which, like the air element, has the characteristics of lightness and motility), then what does that?

In terms of the sequence of treatment for a heat disorder that may manifest as a fever, one must first calm the heat disorder, then balance the wind humor to ensure that the disease does not spread elsewhere. If one does not know how to treat both the heat disorder and wind imbalance in cases of diseases caused by minute organisms, one's treatment

62. Translator's note: Neither of the terms "virus" or "bacteria" has a correlate in Tibetan, but Dr. Dhonden is familiar with these modern terms from his discussions with Western physicians.

may actually cause the spread of the disease. For example, the surgical removal of a tumor in one area may aggravate the underlying problem so that the cancer proliferates all the more swiftly in other parts of the body. Thus, such partial treatment may do more harm than good.

I believe the present proliferation of the AIDS virus is a product of modern times, even though a precursor of this virus did exist in the past. In the Tibetan medical tradition it is included in the category of sexually transmitted diseases, which is separate from the class of microbial and infectious diseases. I have concluded that a precursor of the AIDS virus, specifically a strain of the herpes virus, first existed in a type of tree called in Tibetan "seshing nama" (*se shing rna ma*),[63] that grows in southeastern Tibet, Burma, Thailand, and southern India. This is probably the lacquer tree, or "lac" tree (*Rhus verniciflua*), used by the Japanese and Chinese to make small bowls and lacquer.

Not long ago, I treated a Tibetan monk who had recently escaped from Chinese-occupied Tibet, where he had been imprisoned in a concentration camp. While there, he and his fellow inmates had been sent out to collect wood in the region of Potramo in southeastern Tibet, where the lac tree is quite common. Following this work detail, round lesions appeared on his skin, which covered his body and oozed blood and pus. When I first diagnosed him, he had been suffering from this affliction for three years. His symptoms appeared to be those of a sexually transmitted disease, but he was celibate and had spent the past five years in a concentration camp. I concluded that he had been infected with the virus for which the lac tree is the host, and after treating him for that for five or six months, he was completely cured. This monk now spends much of his time making butter lamp offerings at the main temple in Dharamsala. In Potramo there are also many monkeys, some of which are kept in horse stables due to the Tibetan belief that their presence helps the horses. These monkeys would also become infected with the virus from this tree and transmit it among themselves sexually.

There are two subspecies of this tree, one having dark and the other light-colored wood, but they have other qualities in common. The ascetics of India would make an elixir by squeezing the fruit of this tree, which is about 1.5 inches in length and shaped like the teat of a mare,

---

63. This is not the same as another plant called "seshing" (*bse shing*, or *Semecarpus anacardium*), which is a vine, rather than a tree.

producing an oily red substance. Tibetan doctors also use that fruit as an antidote for various types of microorganisms in the body including the one responsible for leprosy. Both the Japanese and the Chinese also make remedies from the wood of the lac tree. When preparing the lacquer from this wood, the Japanese have developed ways of processing so that they kill the harmful virus that lives in it. Tibetan physicians use only the juice from the fruit of that tree, and they also know how to process it so that the virus is killed. Then that juice is used to kill other types of harmful microorganisms. If this fruit were not processed in that fashion, instead of killing microorganisms, it would produce more harmful microorganisms. When people come in contact with the flowers or leaves of this tree in the spring, when it is blooming, this virus enters into their bodies. Even when the tree is dry, if one lies down for some time at the base of the tree amidst its roots, the heat from one's body will draw out the virus from the roots, and one will become infected.

If a woman who has become contaminated with this lac tree virus engages in sexual intercourse with a man, he will be infected with it. Moreover, if a well-nourished and otherwise healthy woman infected with this virus engages in sexual intercourse with a man who has not eaten for some time, he can easily be infected; but his resistance is considerably heightened if he has intercourse with her after a full meal. One person may also be infected with this virus just by lying in close proximity to a person only *of the opposite sex* who is infected, even without sexual intercourse. One can also be infected from the vapor rising from the urine of a person who is infected with this virus. Symptoms of this disease include a rash, itching, and small pustules on the skin.

In Tibet, people who became ill with this strain of herpes would take medication, including laxatives and emetics, for six to seven months to rid the body of this virus. Sometimes ancillary treatments would be prescribed as well, including blood-letting, hot baths, and so on. During this period, the patient must entirely abstain from sexual intercourse. Once the body has been cleansed, the illness is gone and the person is no longer contagious.

During the late 1960s and early '70s, I visited various countries in Europe, including Spain, Germany, England, and Italy, and also traveled around North America. During those trips, I encountered many cases of the disease known as herpes, and I learned that many pharmaceutical companies were creating drugs to kill or manage the herpes virus. I believe that as a result of people taking those drugs, the herpes virus mutated into the AIDS virus, making treatment for herpes ineffective in the treatment of AIDS. *The Oral Instruction Tantra* implicitly comments on such treatment when it states, "If one does not know how to treat infectious and microbial diseases effectively, one's remedy may exacerbate the disease."[64] Here is a case of a disease that initially could be transmitted only between the sexes, but once the virus mutated, people of the same sex could infect each other, and it has become a far more virulent type of disease. To the best of my knowledge, AIDS has existed for only about the last twenty-five years, but it was prophesied in various ancient Tibetan medical treatises, which describe its nature and origins.

In Tibet there were cases of a disease very similar to herpes, and this could be cured completely, without causing mutations in the microorganisms. In Tibetan medical practice, a whole sequence of medications must be administered to treat herpes in order to counter each symptom and balance the body as a whole. The medicine prescribed to eradicate the herpes virus is called "great medicine." This is quite expensive, so only two or three pills are prescribed, and during the treatment, the patient is told to sleep with an inch-long bar of silver held between the teeth. Then when the virus rises through the vapor in the mouth and comes in contact with the silver, it turns the silver dark. That prevents any detrimental side-effects from the treatment. Otherwise, this virus might come out the mouth and result in dental problems or hair loss.

A Tibetan aphorism states: "My nickels and dimes were taken by the physician, and my hair has been taken by the wood virus. Now that I am free of that virus, I can do whatever I like." The first phrase refers to the expensive treatment for this strain of herpes, the second refers to the hair loss that may occur during the treatment, and the final phrase refers to the patient's ability to re-engage in sexual activity.

On the basis of reports from AIDS patients (and their physicians) I have treated in Europe and America, I have concluded that Tibetan medicine can help this disease. The same Tibetan medicine that was traditionally used in Tibet to treat the strain of herpes associated with the lac tree has proven effective in treating the herpes that is prevalent in the West today; and I have reason to believe it can also kill the AIDS virus.

---

64. *"Rims dang gnyan gyi sgos bcos ma shes na gnyen po nad kyi grogs su 'gro ba srid."*

Since the virus involved in all three illnesses can be eliminated by the same medicine, I conclude that these viruses are all of the same class and that the AIDS virus is a mutated form of the herpes virus.[65]

As in the case of herpes, AIDS cannot be cured with just one medication for everyone, for this disease manifests in the body in relation to one's own specific humoral constitution. In treating AIDS, one must first identify which humor is particularly out of balance and treat that in preparation for the main treatment. This preparatory treatment varies from one individual to another. After this preliminary phase of the treatment, one administers the "great medicine," which is also used to kill the virus. Once the body has been cleansed of this virus, it tends to be quite weak and depleted. So in order to restore the body from the effects of the virus (even though the virus itself has gone), further medication is prescribed in relation to the humoral constitution of the patient. Moreover, an AIDS patient must also refrain from sexual intercourse for six months during this treatment. This disease can be cured only with such individual, multi-phased treatment, but when it is so treated, it does not recur.

To give one example from my own experience of treating this disease, during my stay in New York City in 1996, a young man, probably in his thirties, came to me for a consultation, even though he was in excellent health. I assumed he was coming for a general check-up. But then he reported that in 1989, he had come to me for consultation with two companions, and all three of them had AIDS. At that time, I prescribed medication for all of them, and this man had taken the medication over the course of five years, exactly as I instructed. After those five years had passed, he went to his personal physician to see how he was doing, and his doctor informed him he had no AIDS. He did not believe it, so he went to another doctor, who also diagnosed him as being free of the AIDS virus, and a third doctor told him the same thing. Finally he accepted their diagnosis. His two companions who had also come to me

---

65. Translator's note: Dr. Michael Bachmann, who has devoted years to scientific AIDS research at Stanford University and elsewhere, and who attended these lectures by Dr. Dhonden, commented that the herpes virus and the AIDS virus are very different, so it is scientifically implausible that one is a mutation of the other. As H. H. the Dalai Lama emphasized in his address at the First International Congress on Tibetan Medicine in Washington DC, all Tibetan medical theories, like any scientific theory, should be put to the empirical test.

for treatment had not taken the medication and behavioral advice I gave them, and they had died. I do not recall having treated this person in 1989, for it is not the Tibetan custom to keep long-term records of all one's patients; so I am simply relying on this person's own account.

To give another example, in 1988, while I was visiting Los Angeles, two elderly men phoned from Seattle, saying they were ill and requesting a consultation. At that time the United States government was cracking down on Chinese doctors who were treating AIDS, so I thought these men might be government agents trying to trap me; but I agreed to see them anyway. I was about to fly back to New York at 1:00 on a Sunday afternoon, so I gave them an appointment for 12:30. I figured if they wanted to harass me, they would have to follow me to New York. They arrived just when I was on the verge of leaving for the airport, and they insisted they needed a full consultation. They then reported that in 1986 they had received medication from me for AIDS. I was immediately suspicious, because I had never been to Seattle, so I thought they were setting a trap for me. When I pointed out to them that I had never been to Seattle, they responded that they did not meet me there, but in 1986 they had met me in Colorado, where I had been hosted by a medical doctor named Dr. Weber. They then reported that they were well on their way to recovery, but they both had a lingering cough, and they asked me to give them medication to cure that. Since I do not keep long-term records of all the patients I have seen, I cannot confirm that I actually treated these two people when they said I did. So once again I am relying on others' accounts.

Chapter Thirteen

A Tibetan Medical View of Cancer

Various types of cancer originate from microorganisms, but not of the sort that live in the lac tree; rather, these organisms exist in the atmosphere and descend to earth because of contaminants introduced into the atmosphere, as I discussed earlier. But there is a parallel between the AIDS virus and the organisms responsible for cancer. Both interact with the smallest red organisms, which I mentioned earlier, that are native to the body. When the body is in a state of balance, the three humors are free of the states of excess, deficiency, and disturbance, so they contribute to good health; but when the humors are imbalanced, they contribute to illness. Similarly, when these smallest organisms function on their own, they support the functioning of the body. But when they are attacked by harmful organisms from the external environment—whether those from the lac tree or from the atmosphere—they contribute to illness.

According to Tibetan medicine, there is no one medication that provides effective treatment for all types of cancer. A physician must know how all three humors are involved in the occurrence of any type of cancer, for there may be an imbalance of one, two, or all three humors. Especially when the cancer involves an imbalance of wind or bile—which makes the cancer especially dangerous—it is not enough simply to treat the organisms responsible for the cancer. Therefore, at least three types of medicine must be prescribed to treat the disorder as a whole, and these depend on the humors and elements involved.[66]

---

66. Generally, cancer, such as breast cancer, was quite rare in Tibet. One of the differences between customs of Tibetan and Western women is that when a Tibetan

In India I have encountered many cases of cancer of the large and small intestine, for which medicines were prescribed by Indian doctors that had a cooling effect on the patients' bodies. Sometimes these medications would be administered in combination with the surgical removal of the cancer. However, ingesting such cooling medicines often created a phlegm imbalance, which caused the cancer to re-emerge in the lungs, and then it must be treated all over again. Over the past few decades, I have treated many people in India for lung cancer. If the patient combines Tibetan medicine with surgery, it is especially important for the Tibetan doctor to identify the humoral constitution of the patient; otherwise it is very difficult to bring about a complete cure.

In India I have also encountered many cases of leukemia and liver cancer, for which Tibetan treatment is different than that for other types of cancer. For a number of years, I regularly visited the Tata Hospital in Bombay, where I encountered many cases of leukemia and liver cancer. In these cases, I found that these cancers would disappear in one constituent of the body, but then re-emerge in the bone marrow, which is one of the locations of phlegm. Judging by the way the cancer moved in the body, I concluded that the Indian doctors were prescribing medications that had a cooling effect on the patient's body, which led to phlegm and wind disturbances.

India, the birthplace of the Buddha, is the home of an ancient civilization which has developed the medical tradition known as Āyurveda. Some medical doctors in India are now taking a fresh interest in this ancient tradition, especially concerning its explanation of the three humors, and the wind humor in particular. From both Āyurvedic and Tibetan medical perspectives, the wind humor plays an important role in the body in terms of good and poor health. Another crucial factor to consider when treating diseases is the very close interrelationship between the mind and body. Modern Western doctors tend to treat the

---

woman stops suckling her child, she milks her breast to ensure that all of the milk comes out; and I think this practice lowered the rate of breast cancer among Tibetan women. If a Tibetan woman did find a lump forming in her breast, she would go to a doctor for medication and then go to a tantric adept for *mantra*-blessed water, which she would drink. And she might also go to a lama to receive a *mantra* for her to recite. Thus, she would take steps that were purely medical as well as others that work psychologically and spiritually. But this approach sounds alien to the modern Western mind, so I will not elaborate.

body like a machine, in which one isolated part or another may be broken, in which case they try to cure it or remove it, like any other machine part. All too often, they seem to regard these parts as if there were separate and independent, like components of a machine. Modern medicine also seems to view the body as functioning independently of the mind, as if the mind had no causal efficacy of its own. But this, of course, is not the case. There is a very deep interdependence between the mind and body. But apart from these drawbacks, I believe modern medicine is a highly successful medical tradition. It would be all the more effective, however, if it adopted a more holistic understanding of the individual, including the nature of the five elements as they are present in the body, the external environment, and in the interrelationship between the two.

The various types of cancer develop in relation to the predominant humor associated with them. If the cancer is related to phlegm, it grows slowly; if it is related to bile, it grows very fast; and if it is related to wind, it fluctuates between growth and remission. In the case of a phlegm-related cancer, there is little pain and suffering; if it is related to blood and bile, it tends to be very painful; and if it is wind-related, the painful symptoms fluctuate in intensity. In the case of a phlegm-related cancer, one may experience discomfort at dusk and in the morning; the painful symptoms of a bile-related cancer tend to be more prominent at noon and at midnight; and the symptoms of a wind-related cancer tend to occur in the evening and at dawn. Phlegm-related cancer tends to be aroused chiefly in the spring; bile-related cancer is aroused in the fall; and wind-related cancer is aroused in the summer.

According to Tibetan medicine, since cancer is caused by microorganisms, it is very important not to conduct a biopsy unless it is absolutely imperative, for this creates a disturbance in the body that may exacerbate the disease. I would think that given the enormous amount of cancer research already conducted in the West, medical doctors should be able to detect, with a considerable degree of accuracy, whether or not a cancerous growth is present without performing a biopsy. Surely they must have identified other symptoms of the cancer without having to resort to this invasive procedure. Nevertheless, biopsies still seem to be performed routinely as a major part of the diagnosis. When a medical doctor is quite sure that a cancer is present, I believe it would be more effective to administer the appropriate treatments for the cancer, such as chemotherapy or radiation, without performing a biopsy. In that case, I believe many forms of cancer could be eliminated using modern medical procedures within two or three months. Performing a biopsy has the disadvantage of creating a disturbance that may cause the disease to spread. This is my opinion based on the Tibetan medical tradition, but of course medical doctors have their own rationale for performing biopsies so frequently.

The Tibetan medical tradition is based on the teachings of the Buddha, who is able to see into the future. He has prophesied the nature, origins, and appropriate treatment for various illnesses that are prevalent now. In contrast, modern medicine is based upon scientific research, and it places its hopes in future research, rather than in the authorities from the past. I feel that if medical researchers would focus carefully on the mind-body relationship, they would more deeply understand the nature of illnesses and treat them more effectively.

According to the Buddhist prophecies mentioned earlier, modern illnesses caused by microorganisms—including the various types of cancer and so forth—arise due to contaminants that have been introduced into the atmosphere and the environment at large. To repeat, I believe that atomic and nuclear weapons and many other chemical contaminants including pesticides, herbicides, and many food additives, have contributed to this environmental contamination. I hope Western food does not contribute too much to these diseases, for I have been eating it off and on for more than twenty-five years! Nevertheless, according to the Buddhist tradition, many of these food additives are responsible for many of the modern diseases that beset us now.

I would like to emphasize that the Tibetan medical tradition is based primarily upon the teachings, including the prophesies, of the Buddha, rather than on the research of living Tibetan physicians. Consequently, as we practicing Tibetan doctors diagnose and treat illnesses, we are prone to making mistakes. But such mistakes arise due to our limitations, not because of errors on the part of the Buddha. As a Buddhist, I believe the Buddha had infallible insights into the origins of past and present diseases. New types of medication need to be prepared as antidotes for unprecedented types of diseases caused by microorganisms in this century. This means that we practicing Tibetan doctors must try to understand and produce the medical formulas recorded in ancient manuscripts attributed to the Buddha, for they were not prepared until the corresponding diseases actually appeared. Now that these diseases have become prevalent, these medications must be prepared for the first time, based on formulas written down centuries ago. Moreover, the kinds of diseases that were prevalent in more virtuous eras in the past are now rare. It is also crucial that Tibetan medical students study under the guidance of experienced teachers and physicians in this tradition so that they may learn from the teachers' experience as well as the ancient treatises.

The experiences of one Tibetan physician may differ somewhat from those of others. For example, in addition to the private clinic of the late Dr. Lobzang Dolma and my own private clinic, many Tibetan doctors are treating patients and conducting research in the Tibetan Medical Institute in Dharamsala. This makes Dharamsala the major medical center for the Tibetan community in exile. The specific formulas used in the treatment of liver diseases, cancer, and AIDS differ from one clinic to the another. If a Tibetan doctor has studied very well and fathomed the ancient medical treatises, in addition to serving as an apprentice to a skilled doctor, that is the nature of his or her research. When I first came to India as a refugee in 1959, fleeing from the Communist invasion of Tibet, the responsibility of preserving Tibetan medicine fell largely on my shoulders. In addition to teaching Tibetan medicine to young Tibetans to ensure the tradition was preserved, I also served as the personal physician of the Dalai Lama and his two tutors as well as many other lamas. In addition, I was running a clinic and treating many other patients, and in the process I gained a considerable amount of experience. Over the past few decades of practicing medicine, I have of course observed whether or not specific treatments I was administering were effective, and this has affected how I have prepared medical compounds. So in a way this has constituted a type of research as well, and such research accounts for the differences in medical formulas prepared in the various Tibetan medical clinics.

As for the variety of medical compounds in the Tibetan tradition, there are many medicines for wind disorders, including those known as agar 6, agar 8, agar 15, agar 17, agar 20, agar 25, agar 31, and agar 35. The numbers here indicate the number of ingredients in each compound. To treat the same illness, one doctor may choose one of these, say agar 30 or agar 20, whereas another doctor might prescribe two other wind medications. Some doctors generally prefer one or more of these medications over the others. Likewise, many Tibetan doctors prescribe a single medicine for a specific heat disorder, whereas I will usually prescribe two, for I have found that the interaction between them is more effective. To give another example, a patient may have a strong excess of wind together with a heat disorder related to the blood and bile. In this case some doctors will prescribe one type of medication to be taken in the morning and another in the evening. My preference is to compound these two medications into a single pill so they are taken simultaneously. This custom is also based on certain Tibetan medical classics, so I did not simply make this up on my own. Because of the wide range of Tibetan medical literature, a Tibetan doctor has considerable freedom to choose which ones to draw on in order to maximize the efficacy of his or her treatment.

According to the ancient Tibetan medical tradition, there are three procedures to treat the class of eighteen microbial and infectious diseases. One of these entails the cultivation of meditative concentration (*samādhi*) and the application of this heightened awareness to healing the patient.[67] The second procedure entails the recitation of *mantras,* and the third procedure involves administering herbal medication. Nowadays, there are few Tibetan physicians who are adept in meditative concentration. Some physicians, including myself, do recite therapeutic *mantras* in addition to preparing and dispensing medication.

In cases in which all three of those procedures have been implemented, this has definitely proven effective, especially in cases of infectious diseases. In my experience in India, there are sometimes epidemics of infectious diseases such as influenza. To counteract these, a Tibetan doctor may dispense a medical compound literally called "protection from infection," which has been blessed and empowered with *mantras.* I used to prepare this medicine myself. It is prepared in the form of a large pill, which is wrapped in cloth and is constantly worn around the neck like an amulet as long as one is in a region where such an epidemic is present. When waking up in the morning, the person wearing it sniffs the pill a couple of times and then continues wearing it. On many occasions this has protected people from becoming infected. The efficacy of this medicine stems from the medical ingredients as well as the *mantras* and other influences.

---

67. Translator's note: For a clear, experiential account of methods for developing meditative concentration, see Gen Lamrimpa, *Calming the Mind: Tibetan Buddhist Teachings on Cultivating Meditative Quiescence,* trans. B. Alan Wallace (Ithaca: Snow Lion, 1995).

There is evidence for the efficacy of medical substances in conjunction with the recitation of *mantras*. For example, if a person has been bitten, or suspects he has been bitten, by a rabid dog, a Tibetan physician will ask specific questions about the characteristics of the dog, including its color, and the time when the person was bitten. The patient's responses to these questions will influence which types of medication are prescribed. If the disease has progressed to the point that the patient is mentally imbalanced, the physician or an accomplished Vajrayāna practitioner writes down certain *mantras* on a piece of paper, rolls it up, and recites *mantras* over a volume of water. The water is then empowered with the *mantra*. Then the *mantra*-inscripted paper is given to the rabid person to swallow and then wash down with the water that has been empowered with the *mantra*. This is done early in the morning, when the deranged patient is wobbly on his feet, and the doctor helps the patient to take about fifty steps, during which the patient is told to hold his breath. The doctor makes sure he does not breathe at all, so that no breath escapes from either the mouth or the nose. After taking those fifty steps, the doctor takes out a bell-metal mirror and tells the patient to say "Ha," expelling the breath very rapidly onto the mirror. This is done two or three times. The vapor from the patient's breath appears on the mirror, and, in some cases, a little image of a dog appears in the vapor on the mirror. If so, this indicates that the rabies has been cured, and the person then recovers completely. If no image of a dog appears and the bell metal turns a little dark, this indicates a persistence of the poisoning in the patient's body, in which case medication has to be administered. But no medication is needed if the image of the dog appears, for the disease has been purified by the *mantras* on the slip of paper and in the *mantra*-empowered water.

This treatment for rabies is still in use today, but the above protection from infectious diseases—which is effective only for certain types of infectious diseases such as the flu and the common cold—is not used much any more.

Chapter Fourteen

Benign and Malignant Tumors

Although I have mentioned cancer as a class of diseases due to microorganisms, not all kinds of tumors originate from this cause, for some are simply due to such factors as unhealthy diet and behavior. Tumors known as *trän* (*skran*) belong to the broad classification of serious chronic diseases. I shall now discuss (I) the causes leading to the formation of tumors, (II) the types of diseases within the class of serious chronic diseases, (III) their locations within the body, and (IV) their symptoms. This discussion will pertain to all manner of tumors, of which there is a wide variety.

(I) Serious chronic diseases essentially arise due to inadequate digestion. When the digestive bile is not functioning properly, this also impairs the functioning of the fire-accompanying wind, and this may lead to such diseases. These diseases may arise due to phlegm, blood, or bile; or they may arise due to wind, but due to a disturbance of wind alone. They may also arise due to microorganisms, undigested nutriment, or the ingestion of hair, which directly impairs the digestive bile and indirectly hampers the fire-accompanying wind. Moreover, serious chronic diseases may arise due to demonic influences, but their principal cause is one's previous *karma*. Other causes of such diseases include (1) improper circulation of the blood, such that it accumulates excessively in some parts of the body, leaving other parts relatively depleted; (2) a disturbance of any of the bodily constituents; and (3) blood from wounds inflicted by weapons, such as bullets, spears, and knives. A Tibetan physician will immediately sew up a wound in which the skin is perforated by any such weapons, though if some of the tainted blood from the wound is retained that could cause a serious chronic disease. Diseases of this sort may also arise from the birthing process if some of the woman's uterine blood or any of the placenta or the umbilical cord remains inside her body. Finally, frequently lying on moist ground, especially while wearing inadequate clothing (e.g., sunbathing on wet grass), can lead to serious chronic illnesses, including kidney problems and prostate cancer.

(II) Within the class of great chronic diseases, there are eleven types of tumors, but that classification can be simplified to tumors associated with a heat disorder and those associated with a cold disorder. A more detailed subclassification of these tumors includes twenty types, but I shall not go into those now. (1) The first type of tumor forms in the stomach as a result of indigestion. (2) The second forms due to residue from the blood. In this case, the nutriment from the blood transforms into the flesh, while the residue of the blood goes to the gall bladder. In the gall bladder another segregation should occur, but when that phase of the digestive process is impaired, this can give rise to tumors either in the gall bladder or the small intestine. (3) The next type of tumor, called a "wind tumor," forms in the large intestine, but these tumors do not arise solely due to an imbalance of wind. Rather, they arise due to a disturbance of wind in dependence on some other factor, such as the serous fluid, phlegm, improper digestion, or the ingestion of hair, as mentioned earlier. That is called a "wind tumor," because it forms in the large intestine, which is a principal location of wind. (4) The next type of tumor is called a "blood tumor," for it forms inside the uterus in dependence on the blood, and there are five subclasses of this type of tumor. Tumors are also classified with regard to their location, namely, (5) the outer, (6) inner, or (7) mid-region of the body. They are also subclassified with regard to their association with (8) wind, (9) bile, and (10) phlegm. Finally, as mentioned earlier, tumors are classified according to their association with (11) heat and cold disorders.

(III) Wind tumors arise in the large intestine, and bile tumors occur only in the gall bladder or the small intestine. Another type of tumor that arises due to inadequate functioning of the decomposing phlegm occurs in the stomach and the large intestine. Tumors associated with a blood disorder predominantly occur in the liver, spleen, or the uterus, but on rare occasions they may form in the stomach or the large intestine.

In terms of the locations of the outer, inner, and mid-regions of the body, the outer regions include the exterior of the body as a whole, especially the skin, and the outer areas of the hollow organs. The inner regions of the body include the interior of the hollow and solid organs. The mid-regions of the body include the interior surfaces of the hollow organs and the mid-regions of the solid organs, as opposed to their periphery or center.

(IV) In terms of symptoms, the first type of tumor is called a "food tumor," for it arises due to indigestion, especially in the first phase of the digestive process, in which mucus accumulates in the stomach, impairing the segregation of the nutriment from the residue. Such tumors form principally in the stomach.

Another type of cancer forms due to impaired liver functioning, entailing bleeding from the liver. Like a clay pot that has not be properly baked, the liver "leaks" blood, which may go into the small intestine. Normally some bile flows from the gall bladder into the small intestine and passes out with the feces and urine. However, when the bile that goes into the small intestine from the gall bladder joins with the blood being secreted from the liver, tumors may form in the small intestine. This is because the heat of the bile mixing with the blood, resulting in a very tough tumor that forms in the small intestine.

The next type of tumor is associated with the three phases of the digestive process in the stomach involving the decomposing phlegm, the digestive bile, and the fire-accompanying wind. As a result of this three-fold digestive process, the nutriment goes to the liver. However, if the liver is not functioning properly, the further segregation of nutriment from residue that should take place in the liver does not occur. Consequently, both the inadequately processed residue and nutriment pass on to the gall bladder, resulting in an accumulation of the residue and nutriment in the gall bladder. This can result in either the formation of gall stones or tumors in the gall bladder. This disorder in the gall bladder may also be carried by the wind humor to the stomach, the large intestine, and especially the uterus and ovaries.

Another type of tumor fluctuates in size, first growing large, then going into remission, and then growing again. This fluctuation is due to wind, which also moves them around in the body. If such a patient is given proper medication, such wind tumors can be cured quickly. Recall, once again, that such tumors form not solely due to a wind imbalance, but in relationship to some other constituent of the body such as the serous fluid, phlegm, blood, or bile. Because of its light and motile nature, wind by itself cannot cause a tumor.

As mentioned earlier, tumors may form in the uterus as a result of the retention of blood following the birthing process. The blood needs to be flushed out completely. Such tumors are relatively easy for a Tibetan physician to identify, but then one must make a further diagnosis to determine whether the tumor is malignant or benign.

Microorganisms are responsible for some types of tumors, but not for all. Malignant tumors, which are presently so common in the West, do originate from microorganisms. Tumors that form in the liver and the gall bladder are associated with a heat disorder, and in cases where they are produced by microorganisms, they commonly move elsewhere in the body, such as the brain.

As I explained earlier, cancer is included among the eighteen types of microbial and infectious diseases, which are further classified into forty diseases. The Tibetan term "hlokpa" (*lhog pa*) refers to a type of microorganism and to the disease due to that organism. The symptoms of this disease include a single massive, painful, red swelling on the limbs, throat, or anywhere else in the body. In the Tibetan tradition this is treated with medication, and a Buddhist tantric practitioner may also recite *mantras*. A combination of herbal medication and *mantra* recitation is also used when the inflammation bursts and emits fluid and a small lump of flesh, about the size of an eyeball. According to Tibetan custom, this lump of flesh is removed and washed, and then the patient is told to swallow it. This acts like an inoculation, so the patient will be immune to that kind of disease in the future. While growing up in nomad country in Tibet, I witnessed this many times, and it seemed to prevent the recurrence of that disease.

The *hlokpa* organism comes from livestock, and in Tibet it came solely from bovine creatures, including male and female yaks,[68] cattle, and *dzo*, which are a cross between a bull and a female yak. When one of these animals would die, Tibetans would skin it and while doing so, the *hlokpa* organism could be transmitted from the animal's flesh through the skin to the flesh of the skinner. People who were so infected and who received

---

68. Translator's note: In Tibetan only the male of this species is called a yak (*g.yag*), while the female is called a dri (*'bri*).

proper treatment would then swallow the lump of flesh, as I mentioned, and that made them immune to this disease thereafter, even if they were infected again. However, those who did not receive proper treatment would die from this disease, and their corpses would then becomes a source of infection for others.

Strangely enough, it was not contagious from one human body to another until after the first person had died. This being known in Tibet, when disposing of such a corpse, people would make sure that they did not touch the corpse. Rather, when they took it to the cremation grounds, they would wrap it on poles and carry it at a distance from their own bodies. I believe that if such a growth were lanced or surgically removed, it would form a scab that would continue to emit pus and other fluids, and it would become incurable, for the causal microorganism would still be present. In Tibet people infected with this disease who perforated the swelling or tried to cut it out might live for quite a few years, but the swelling remained, with a little hole in it that would continually ooze serous fluid and pus.

The above account of the Tibetan way of treating this disease is drawn from my own experience, for I grew up among nomads and saw this done. I saw for myself what worked and what did not, and this mode of treatment was common knowledge among the nomadic people of Tibet. I suspect that when great herds of buffalo used to roam freely in America, that same type of microorganism was probably present and could transmit that disease.

Tibetan nomads living on the northern plateau of Tibet roved around, especially in the summer, staying in one place for a month while letting their livestock graze, and then moving on to another place for a month at a time. These people had the best practical knowledge of this particular type of disease. Nomads in that region and in southern Tibet where I grew up would observe the place where one of their animals died, and they would later watch the area around the carcass when it had snowed. If the beast had been free of this organism, the snow around it would not melt; but if it had been infected, the snow would melt due to the presence of that organism. If the nomads found that the snow had melted for this reason, they would build a little wall of dried yak dung around the infected carcass. Then they would set fire to this wall of dried yak dung, which would remain burning for three to five days. In that way they made sure the microorganism was completely eliminated so it would not spread elsewhere. When the fire died all the way down, they would observe markings on the ground around the carcass that indicated the former presence of this organism.

When I was growing up, my family owned six to seven hundred head of yak and cattle and around three thousand sheep. Even small households owned two thousand sheep. When I was six or seven years old and was living in the south of Tibet, a couple of men became infected with this disease. One of them noticed the swelling and immediately consulted a doctor, took medication, and was completely cured. Years later I went to Lhasa to study medicine, and when I eventually returned home, I met this fellow and saw that he had a lot of scar tissue on the side of his neck where that lump of flesh had emerged and then healed over. That was the only remaining sign of that disease. The other person tried to cure himself by lancing the boil-like protrusion, but he died. His neighbors recognized the cause of his death, and they warned me to stay away from his corpse. To dispose of the corpse, they sought out people who had been infected with that disease and had acquired immunity in the way I described previously.

A couple of hours' walk away from my home was a region that had been widely infected with this organism. A lot of livestock died there, so that area was abandoned by the nomads, for none of them wanted to graze their livestock there. To discover where these organisms were still present in the soil, even in the absence of livestock, they waited for a big snowstorm, and then looked for areas in the snow that had melted due to that organism. Once those spots were identified, they constructed walls of dried yak dung surrounding the infected areas, and set them ablaze. These fires smoldered for about ten days. When examining one spot after the fire had burned itself out, we found a fist-sized charred lump of flesh with a lot of markings on it like little eyes. We never did understand why it was marked like that.

This *hlokpa* disease is one of the eighteen types of microbial and infectious diseases. Such organisms initially form in the atmosphere, penetrate the body, and then join with the small, red organisms that are native to the human body. There are seven types of these airborne organisms.

The various types of cancer that form in the brain, liver, lungs, and so forth, are not included in the type of tumor known in Tibetan as *trän*, which are generally benign, but rather in the class of microbial and infectious diseases. I shall first discuss the types of small organisms—especially those that appear on the exterior of the body—that can be seen with the naked eye. These organisms enter the body from the atmosphere, invade the blood stream, and thereby spread throughout the body. This infection leads to a heat disorder that may then descend upon the right and left sides of the throat and upon the right and left sides of the back of the neck. Then it may spread to the temples, the front of the armpits, the left and right sides of the waist at the level of the kidneys, the left and right sides of the lower abdomen at the level of the small intestine, and the left and right sides of the groin. It spreads only on the surface of the body, not the inner organs. It most commonly occurs on the left and right front of the neck, the temples, and the left and right sides of the groin.

There are many types of disorders that descend on these surface areas of the body, and they are distinguished in terms of their coloration, tough or pliant consistency, their degree of heat, the rate of their maturation, and their growth or remission. Various types of symptoms are to be examined in this regard. This class of disease may arise in relation to disorders of the wind, bile, phlegm, blood, flesh, fat, or the channels. One may also develop certain types of inflammation or lesions on the surface of the skin, and if these become infected, they may also lead to this class of disease. When such an organism first invades the body, it gives rise to a heat disorder, the symptoms of which are chills, shivering, and aching and discomfort throughout the body. Even though there is much heat in the body, one still feels cold, regardless of how much clothing one puts on. These are the initial symptoms of a heat disorder due to such an infection, and that later ripens and spreads in the body as mentioned previously. In fact, these symptoms are very similar to those of the common cold or the flu, and to the initial symptoms of smallpox and chicken pox. According to the Tibetan tradition, there are various types of chicken pox, which are classified by the colors white, red, and multicolored. There is also a strain of chicken pox to which children are especially prone. Even these types of pox are included in the general classification of forty microbial and infectious diseases.

Among the class of eighteen microbial and infectious diseases, most are prophesied to occur only during the degenerate era of the last five hundred years of the Buddha's teachings, but there is one that has been around for a long time. This is a complex and very serious disorder due to a combination of three factors. The first is a type of microorganism; the second is the influence of non-human creatures called *nāgas*, which can be aroused by digging in the earth, polluting bodies of water, and so on; and the third is one's own *karma*. Although this disease has been present for a long time, it is especially prevalent in this century. This disease, known as leprosy, was rare in ancient times, at least in Tibet, but now, due to the present degenerate era, it has become more prevalent.

In the Tibetan medical tradition, cancers are included in two classes of diseases: the thirty-two (or more extensively, the forty) classes of women's disorders, such as breast tumors, and the class of eighteen microbial and infectious disorders.

Women are subject to nine types of tumors, not all of which are cancerous, which may generally occur anywhere in the body, though in women they are more prevalent in the ovaries, the uterus, and the breasts.

(1) The first of these, which is not very dangerous, even though it may appear quite large when examined with an x-ray, is called a "bubbly tumor of the uterus." It forms due to a mixing of menstrual blood and serous fluid, conjoined with an unsteady menstrual cycle, with a large menstrual flow some months and a small flow in other months. This can be easily cured with a small amount of medicine.

(2) The second type of tumor, which is related to the menstrual blood, is called a "firm blood tumor."[69] Such tumors form in the uterus (and ovaries) as a result of an incomplete evacuation of the menstrual blood, and they may grow so large it looks as if the woman is pregnant. Such tumors are very firm and are difficult to cure. Their symptoms including fluctuating (from acute to mild) pain in the small intestine.

(3) The third kind of tumor, called an "insensitive tumor of the flesh," forms into firm, insensitive lumps that are not painful when pressed or prodded. This slow-forming tumor appears in the uterus, the ovaries, and the fallopian tubes. Its symptoms include acute pain in the waist region, as if the hip bones were broken, discomfort on both sides of the ilium and on the lower back side of the ischium, indigestion, blockage of the urinary tract, and a bloated sensation in the stomach, as if air from the stomach were ascending.

---

69. Translator's note: *khrag skran hrem po*. All nine of these tumors are explained in the three-volume treatise *Bod kyi gso rig slob deb*, by Blo bzang bstan 'dzin (Dharamsala: Bod gzhung sman rtsis khang gso rig mtho slob sde tshan), Vol. III, pp. 375-378.

(4) The fourth type of tumor, called a cystoid tumor, forms in the interior and exterior of the vagina. Its symptoms include difficulty in urination, a burning sensation when urinating, dark menstrual blood, reduced menstrual flow, weight loss, fluctuating pain, and a feeling of heaviness in the lower portion of the body.

(5) The fifth tumor is a stomach tumor that occurs specifically in women. Symptoms of this tumor include a loss of strength in the lower portion of the body from the hips down, a sense of heaviness that alternatingly moves from the right hip and thigh to the left hip and thigh, discomfort in the heart, shortness of breath, and a sense of fullness of breath as if one's respiration were disrupted, and a sense of malaise or depression. Even though this is called a stomach tumor, it occurs far more prevalently in the uterus, with only about one percent of instances of this tumor occurring in the stomach.

(6) The sixth type of tumor is called "a dark residual tumor." Following the birthing process, if some of the tissue, placenta, serous fluid, and blood are retained inside the woman, this may cause a tumor. Such tumors are called "residual" due to these retained substances. According to Tibetan custom, for a week after a woman gives birth, she remains warm in bed, eats well, relaxes, and sleeps a great deal. By so doing, if her body is retaining any residual blood or serous fluid, it will gradually be completely secreted, and this prevents the formation of this type of tumor. Symptoms of this tumor include darkening of the complexion and swelling and discomfort in the joints. It is very easy to mistake this disorder for rheumatoid arthritis.

(7) The seventh type of tumor is called "a dangling tumor of the channels," for such tumors "dangle" in the fallopian tubes. In cases of a long and painful birthing process, the midwife may forcibly draw the infant from the womb, and this can cause such a tumor. A caesarean operation may also lead to this type of tumor. In either of those two situations, the fallopian tubes may be damaged, and it is this that causes the formation of a tumor.

Five years ago, I encountered a Tibetan woman living in India who had had a caesarean operation, after which she continued to emit fluids. Two more operations were performed, but the problem was still not identified and her illness continued. Eventually she consulted me, and I asked to see her sister and father as well, while her husband had already emigrated to the United States. I examined her and discovered this type of tumor in her fallopian tubes. I then suggested to her, "Before I treat you, ask your lama for a divination to see whether you should go to the hospital in Kangra, in Ludhiāna, or in Chandīgarh. If the divination indicates that you should go either to Ludhiāna or Chandīgarh, you should have x-rays taken and then show them to me. If the divination indicates that you should go to the hospital in Kangra, follow the advice of the doctor there, but let me know what he says." The reason for this final request was that Kangra is very close to Dharamsala, where I live, and I had worked in close collaboration with the doctors there. The woman then followed my suggestion and consulted her *lama,* Dema Lochö Rinpoche, who agreed to perform this divination. It indicated that she should go to the hospital in Kangra. Before taking an x-ray, the doctors there asked about my diagnosis. I told them that my pulse and urine analysis indicated there was a blockage in her fallopian tubes—possibly caused by filaments of a cotton swab left from one of her operations—in addition to a tumor of this sort.

The doctors at the Kangra hospital then took x-rays and detected an obstruction in the fallopian tubes. They then performed another surgery and removed a tumor from her fallopian tubes about the size of the tip of a thumb. This was a significant accomplishment in this small-town hospital, and they filmed the entire procedure. After her operation, the woman came back to me, and I gave her medication to complete her recovery. Her health was finally fully restored, and she is presently living in the United States, I believe. The doctors who had treated her previously were rather embarrassed at this outcome, for this tumor formed due to their previous surgeries. The father of this woman took legal action against them, which resulted in their returning the 40,000 rupees they had charged her for the previous operations. This was then offered to His Holiness the Dalai Lama.

(8) The eighth tumor, called an "ovum tumor," forms when the ovum and the semen unite. Due to improper diet or conduct or to defective semen, the embryo does not develop, and the resultant putrefaction of the union of semen and ovum can give rise to a tumor. Symptoms of this type of tumor include an increased frequency of menstrual flow, such that it occurs every week or two, a feeling of unhappiness, general discomfort throughout the body, and aching of the muscles and bones.

(9) The final type of tumor is called a "*zaku* blood tumor." The term *zaku* refers to healthy blood. During menstruation, the type of blood that should flow is called residual blood, and it should be evacuated from the body. But in some cases, together with this blood, normal healthy blood also flows out, and this can lead to the formation of this type of tumor. In this case, the ovum comes from the ovaries down into the uterus and remains there, but since the menstrual blood is not flowing properly, more blood flows into the uterus and accumulates there. This leads to the formation of a tumor in the uterus that can grow so large it appears as if the woman is pregnant. Symptoms of this tumor include abdominal distention and discomfort and morgarigamy.

Another type of woman's disorder entails the arousal of microorganisms that are native to the uterus. This is another type of tumor not included in the above class of nine tumors in women or the class of eighteen microbial and infectious diseases. Its symptoms include discomfort in the front and back of the ilia, vaginal itching, attentional instability, insomnia, restlessness, and a foul odor emitted from the urinary tract. Most tumors that form in the uterus do not belong to the class of microbial and infectious diseases. However, tumors that form in the breasts and lymph nodes are included in that category. One indication that they are caused by microorganisms is that further tumors often form after the initial ones are surgically removed from the lymph nodes or breasts. Although this is a type of microbial disease, it is not infectious.

When an experienced oncologist performs a diagnosis and concludes that a tumor is probably malignant, I believe, as I mentioned earlier, that it is best to proceed immediately to treatment—be it surgery, chemotherapy, radiation, or a combination of those treatments—without performing a biopsy. Even if the tumor turns out to be benign, the patient will largely recover from the above forms of treatment. But by perforating a tumor, a biopsy tends to cause cancer to spread in the body, especially when the tumor occurs in the breast or lymph nodes. My own preference would be to apply radiation and chemotherapy first; then, after the tissue is dead, it may be surgically removed without causing the cancer to spread.

Over the years that I practiced medicine in Tibet, I treated many women suffering from a wide variety of disorders. I never encountered any cases of breast cancer. Sometimes a lump would form in the breast, which was attributed to influences by *nāgas,* and for this a woman would go to a *lama* to receive a spiritual practice to counteract *nāgas*, and to a doctor to receive medication. In some cases the lump would burst and pus would emerge from it, and then it would heal. In other cases it would not burst, but it could be completely healed with proper medication.

I have also treated women with this disorder in India. In one case about ten years ago, a woman patient of mine developed a large lump in her breast. An Indian medical doctor told her she had breast cancer. She then consulted me, and I suggested that she ask her *lama* to perform a divination to determine what kind of non-human influences might have contributed to her problem and how those entities might be appeased through spiritual practice. In addition, I first gave her a salve to be placed on the breast in order to retract the illness there. Then I gave her another salve to apply to the breast at the same spot in order to open up the lump and draw out the pus. This is done without lancing it. For the final phase of treatment, I applied a dough of parched barley meal as a salve to gently draw out any residual pus in this wound. As a result of this treatment, she fully recovered and is alive and well today.

I have been practicing medicine in India since 1961, and during this time I have treated many women. Breast tumors are relatively uncommon among Tibetan women, but in most cases when they have come to me with this problem, I have simply prescribed medication and given them advice on their diet and behavior. This has usually been enough to effect a complete cure. Over these years, I have encountered only two or three cases of malignant breast cancer among Tibetan women and only four or five instances among the many Indian women I have treated. But over the course of my many visits to Europe and North America, I have treated many cases of breast cancer.

I believe the reason why breast cancer is so rare among Tibetan women is that in Tibet women would traditionally breastfeed their children for three or four years, or in some cases for as long as six or seven years. This is a healthy practice that prevents breast cancer. In the West, many women do not breastfeed their infants at all, or they do so for only a short time; and I believe that is one cause of breast cancer.

Questions and Responses

QUESTION: There is some discussion in the West these days about the pros and cons of giving immunizations. What is your opinion of giving inoculations and other types of immunization?

RESPONSE: For my medical practice and views, I simply rely upon the teachings of the Buddha, including *The Four Tantras* and so forth. I am not clairvoyant, and I have no great contemplative realizations, so it is difficult for me to have an informed opinion on this matter. Traditional Tibetan treatment that results in life-long immunity to smallpox, for instance, is directly applied to the channel associated with the lungs.

When people in traditional Tibet became infected with smallpox, they would be placed in quarantine. In addition, such people would be given no meat, alcohol, or sweet foods that would exacerbate this illness. Once the smallpox matures and the head of the pustules becomes dark, the patient would be given medication for a wind disorder and some meat to eat, and that would cure the disease. After they were healed, the dried up skin from the pox would be gathered, dried, and ground up into a fine powder. This powder mixed with medication would then be used as preventative medication for people who had not been infected. A small amount of the powder would be applied to the skin on the inside of the wrist where the lung channel runs, and it would be bound there with apricot skin. Eventually a fairly large (one-half inch in diameter), pale pustule would form at that place, and the person would experience a fever, though the pustule itself would not be very painful. If this was properly done, only one pustule would form; otherwise a few would appear. When that pustule dried up and healed, a doctor would remove its scab, make a powder of it, and that would be used to immunize others. The powder from such a scab acts as the most potent type of inoculation.

This kind of inoculation would also be used by nomads on their livestock. Some virulent strains of infectious diseases would kill two to three hundred of their yak and cattle at a time. Nomads experienced in such matters would draw some blood from one of the diseased animals before it died, and they would keep it warm, without letting the warmth of the blood dissipate. Then they would mix this with an herbal medication, and to keep it warm they would put it inside their garments right next to the skin. Then this mixture would be infused into the nostrils of uninfected beasts to inoculate them from that disease. Right now there is a doctor in the Dzoki region of northeastern Tibet who is especially good at this.

QUESTION: Tibetan physicians take an oath not to harm other sentient beings, yet in Tibetan medical treatises there are many references to types of healthy and unhealthy meat for people with different humoral constitutions; and in some cases meat is used in Tibetan medicines. Is there not an inconsistency here?

RESPONSE: It is quite true that a Tibetan physician is to avoid harming sentient beings, and there are indeed many references in Tibetan medical literature to meat-eating. But meat is not used in any Tibetan medicine, although bear musk is sometimes used in minute amounts, and that does entail killing bears. It is said that a Tibetan physician should guard the lives of all creatures, even insects, as if they were his own. On the other hand, a Tibetan doctor may tell a patient what types of meat are healthy and unhealthy for a specific ailment. For example, the patient might be told eat mutton, but the doctor would not order him to butcher a sheep; for in that case both the doctor and the patient would accrue the *karma* of killing. The doctor is simply stating a medical fact that if the patient were to eat mutton this would help the disease. According to Buddhist ethics, if an animal is not killed specifically for oneself, one does not accumulate the *karma* of killing it, even if one eats its flesh. On the other hand, if nobody in a whole community ate meat, then the butchers would be out of a job, and the animals would not be killed. Thus, there is still a misdeed in buying and eating meat, even if one is not directly responsible for killing the animal in question.

To cite another related situation, when my interpreter, Alan Wallace, lived in India for four years in the early 1970s, he eventually became infested with three types of parasites, some of which emerged in his stool. I gave him medication to rid his body of these parasites. As a Tibetan doctor, even though I am to cherish even the smallest of sentient beings, human life has a greater value than that of an intestinal parasite. So even though it is detrimental to kill these worms, since his human life is more valuable, I gave him the medication. In all cases, one must judge where there is greater benefit and where there is greater harm. Because we made the decision as we did, you have Alan as interpreter today. If I had placed a higher priority on the lives of the tapeworms, they would be doing little good for anyone at this point.

QUESTION: Historically, has Tibetan medicine included the practice of autopsy?

RESPONSE: Yes, this has been practiced in Tibet for more than two thousand years. When a person died, the corpse would be opened up so that doctors could get a clear view of its interior. This practice is also discussed in Tibetan medical treatises. Autopsies were still frequently performed when I was a youngster studying in Tibet. In fact, Tibet was the easiest place in the world to do this, due to the Tibetan tradition of chopping up human corpses to feed to the vultures and other wild animals. There was absolutely no stigma or taboo against performing autopsies. There were people in Tibet whose livelihood it was to take corpses to the peaks of mountain and chop them up to make them easier for the vultures to consume. They learned a lot about human anatomy. One exception was the case of infectious diseases, in which there was a prohibition against cutting up corpses in that fashion. It was the law that such contaminated corpses were to be buried, and not cut up or cremated.

Apart from a few high *lamas,* no one was cremated in Tibet. This was not due to a lack of firewood, for many places in Tibet were heavily forested. Rather, Tibetans preferred to give their dead bodies to the vultures as a final gesture of generosity. When a corpse is burned, no one benefits from it. There is an analogous practice in Tibetan Buddhism known as "chö" (*gcod,* literally meaning "to cut"), in which one imagines giving one's body to carnivorous spirits, who may take on the form of vultures.

Chapter Fifteen
Wholesome Behavior

Lifetime Behavior

I shall now address an aspect of preventative medicine, namely the different types of lifetime, seasonal, and occasional behavior to follow in order to remain healthy. This same counsel can be followed in times of illness. Lifetime healthy behavior is of two types: behavior for the pursuit of mundane ends, and behavior for the pursuit of spiritual ends.

Mundane Conduct

Within the category of behavior for the pursuit of mundane ends, there is conduct to promote longevity, including the use of elixirs and what are called "precious pills" and "ambrosial pills" in the Tibetan medical tradition. Precious pills are prepared by a doctor, while ambrosial pills are usually prepared by a highly realized *lama* and are taken as blessings. Precious pills promote longevity. In the Tibetan tradition, there is a common custom of writing down a prayer or *mantra* for longevity, placing this on an altar, and consecrating that inscription with meditation and *mantra* recitation. This is usually done by a *lama*, then the inscribed piece of paper is folded up, placed inside an amulet, and worn around the neck as a talisman.

Another ancient method for promoting longevity and preventing disease is to ingest the medicinal fruit known as the "victorious" type of chebulic myrobalan.[70] However, because of the decrease of merit in the world, this fruit has virtually disappeared. It is said that the fruit of this tree prevents all types of infectious diseases. I have been able to purchase a few of these fruits. The ones I bought were about three inches long, and each one cost roughly $60. One piece of this fruit, when mixed in a single medical compound, does not even make enough medicine to make up one month's prescription.

Other medicinal substances that are both ingested and used in talismans include sweet flag,[71] mustard seed, and the Indian bedellium tree.[72] Other nonmedicinal substances used in talismans include relics, such as ashes or fine, granulated spheres that sometimes appear in the cremated remains of realized beings. Diamonds, lapis lazuli, sapphires, emeralds, "*zee* stones,"[73] now worn as ornaments embedded in gold, were originally used in Tibet as protection from weapons and infectious diseases.

We are presently living in the historical era when the teachings of Buddha Śākyamuni are still extant, as well as relics of his remains, preserved in *stūpas*, or reliquaries, such as the famous Boudhanath *stūpa* in Kathmandu, Nepal. It is said that when the Buddha's teachings completely vanish from our world, all the relics of the *buddhas* and *bodhisattvas* of our era will go into the ocean and there turn into jewels that will be protected by *nāgas*. According to Buddhist lore, all the emeralds, diamonds, and sapphires present today are transmuted relics from earlier enlightened beings. Relics of Buddha Śākyamuni may also be worn as a talisman or placed upon an altar and worshipped. This yields many blessings, as these holy relics continue to serve the needs of sentient beings.

The relics from the body of a *buddha* transform into a wish-fulfilling jewel imbued with fourteen qualities. For example, when such a jewel is

---

70. Translator's note: A lengthy description of the different types of myrobalan is to be found in *The Quintessence Tantras of Tibetan Medicine*, trans. Dr. Barry Clark (Ithaca: Snow Lion, 1995), pp. 148-149.

71. Ibid., p. 151.

72. Ibid., p. 146.

73. These naturally formed, elongated stones with "eyes" on them are extremely prized among Tibetans. The more eyes a stone has, the more valuable it is, with the most expensive ones having nine eyes.

supplicated, it grants all wishes; and it can dispel darkness, cure illness, ward off malevolent spirits, promote longevity, and clear one's complexion. According to Buddhist belief, such wish-fulfilling gems are present in the ocean right now, but they are discovered only during an era in which a virtuous world emperor (*cakravartin*) is in power. When Buddha Śākyamuni was born, it was prophesied that he could either become a world emperor, or he could become a perfectly awakened being, or *buddha*.

The relics of a *bodhisattva* that transform into precious jewels have eleven of the fourteen qualities of the wish-fulfilling jewel that manifests from the relics of a *buddha*. Those of *arhats* (beings who have irreversibly freed themselves from all mental afflictions and the cycle of *saṃsāra*) transform into jewels bearing seven of those qualities. Finally, the relics of other realized beings who have not yet become *buddhas, bodhisattvas,* or *arhats* transform into jewels having five or as few as two of those qualities. Although such relics are in the ocean right now, they can be found only by people with great merit, as narrated in many Buddhist *sūtras*.

The scientific explanation of the origin of diamonds originating from compressed coal is different from the Buddhist view. According to Buddhist legend, the origin of diamonds traces back to a *bodhisattva* named Satyakathāsiddhi, the literal meaning of which is "the adept whose words of truth come true." It is said of this *bodhisattva* that whatever prayers he made came true. Satyakathāsiddhi lived 80,000 years ago, and throughout the five hundred years of his life he completely abstained from killing, and he lived on a diet consisting only of yogurt. When he was about to die, he ascended to the peak of Mount Meru, the mountain in the center of this world according to traditional Buddhist cosmology.

Among the relics from his body, one of his shoulder blades was made into a wheel and the other was made into a spear by the god Viṣṇu. Of these two weapons, legend has it that they infallibly hit their target, and the object struck invariably perishes; but anyone who is killed with them is protected from rebirth in all miserable states of existence. In traditional Tibet, people who had committed great sins, such as murder, would commonly pray to die by being struck with one of these weapons of Viṣṇu. Other bones from Satyakathāsiddhi were made into ornaments by Brahmā and other gods, while yet others were powdered and carried by the wind to Bodhgaya, where they turned into diamonds. The Tibetan name for Bodhgaya is Dorje Den (rDo rje gdan), meaning "the vajra seat," and in this case "*vajra*" means "diamond." Buddhist tradition declares that the thousand *buddhas* of this fortunate eon will attain enlightenment in Bodhgaya.

To return to the topic of longevity, one should avoid the two types of conditions that result in premature death, namely, unwholesome behavior and diet; so one should always be mindful and vigilant to avoid these at all times. Most types of illnesses arise in dependence on one's diet and conduct. Many illnesses occur due to eating many kinds of food together. Even if the individual ingredients of the food are healthy, some combinations are detrimental to the health. Even if one does not detect the illness immediately, it can accumulate gradually and lead to disease over the long term. Moreover, if one travels to a foreign country where the food is different from one's habitual diet, and one eats excessive amounts of this alien food, that too can give rise to illness.

Generally speaking, if any food, especially unfamiliar food, is eaten in excess just for the enjoyment of its taste, it will be detrimental to one's health. Over-consumption of beer, hard liquor, and raw meat and vegetables is unhealthy; but I must add that people who grow up accustomed to unhealthy diets may be able to withstand them better, even if they eat at improper times with respect to the humors. On the other hand, if someone who is not accustomed to eating sweets consumes them in great quantities, this could lead to a phlegm disorder. Over-consumption of astringent or rough foods can give rise to a wind disorder, and a diet that consists principally of oily foods can give rise to a bile disorder. In such cases there are generally two reasons why one falls ill: the first is that one is eating unfamiliar food, and the second is that one is eating at the wrong time.

Unwholesome behavior pertains to one's body, speech, and mind. Unwholesome speech includes words motivated by arrogance, attachment, and hatred, pointless conversation, and all kinds of abuse and disparagement. One who is habituated to such unwholesome speech becomes prone to bile disturbances. To avoid unwholesome mental behavior, one should constantly bear in mind the results of one's deeds, especially in terms of their long-term, ethical consequences. For all types of physical, verbal, and mental activity, it is important not to work to the point of exhaustion, for this too results in illness.

With regard to one's behavior concerning the five types of sensory objects, it is important to experience these in moderation. Some types of unwholesome sensory enjoyments are simply to be avoided, but for the rest one should enjoy them without over-indulgence or extreme abstinence.

The following is traditional, general advice for healthy conduct. While in motion, it is important to watch where one is going, looking backwards and forwards and attending to the surrounding environment. When sitting down on the grass or other surfaces, one should look first, for one may be about to sit on an insect or some other living being and either kill it or be harmed by it. According to Tibetan tradition, which may or may not be applicable in the modern world—when moving around at night, one should go with a companion and carry a stick for protection. When entering unknown territory, one should first discover whether it is frequented by bandits; and if one is traveling through a forest that is on fire, one should travel upwind from the fire and watch out for burning coals under the ash. When hiking in the mountains in the summertime, one should beware of loose rock and sand that may start an avalanche. One should not climb trees in midwinter when the branches may be brittle and encrusted with ice. Whether one is inside or outside, it is important to beware of danger from the environment. For example, in the south of India there are some regions where one must always look out for poisonous snakes. If one must enter a dangerous area, it is important to go with a trustworthy, reliable friend.

It is imperative to sleep during the nighttime. In the West, many people think of the night as a time to party, but they are wrong. It is a time to sleep. If one occasionally sleeps too little at night, one should take a nap the following day. If one allows oneself to become deprived of sleep for a sustained period, this will lead to the accumulation of wind disturbances, which will later be aroused, especially in the summer. Particularly during the early summer, one should get extra rest by taking a nap during the daytime. Moreover, if one has had too little sleep at night due to becoming intoxicated, experiencing great grief, excessive conversation, or because one is advanced in years, it is especially important to make up for it during the daytime.

During the fall and early winter, from October through December, one should not sleep during the daytime, for this may lead to a phlegm disorder and the body may become swollen or even succumb to gout and edema. If one grows accustomed to sleeping in the daytime during those seasons and follows an inappropriate diet, excessive fluid accumulates in the body, making it bloated, the mind becomes dull, and one becomes prone to headaches, lethargy, and colds. If one is afflicted by such a phlegm imbalance, one should either fast or take an emetic. If one is suffering from constant insomnia, one should drink milk, beer, meat broth, and melted butter, and smear sesame oil on the head and inside the ears.

As for sexual conduct, one should abstain from intercourse with any non-human creature, with anyone else's spouse, with a person who is in failing health (indicated by poor complexion, emaciation and so forth), a pregnant woman at any stage of the pregnancy, and a woman during her menstrual period. In terms of the frequency of healthy sexual activity, during the wintertime one can engage in as much sexual activity as one likes; during the fall and spring, one should have sexual intercourse no more frequently than every other day; and during the early and later summer, one should have sexual intercourse no more often than once every fortnight. If one engages in excessive sexual intercourse, one's sense faculties, including one's vision, hearing and even one's intelligence, will become impaired, resulting in dizziness and premature death. There is no minimum amount of healthy sexual activity; in fact, it is best for one's health to remain chaste.

Tibetan medical treatises state that conduct in accordance with societal norms, such as basic courtesy, is the basis for all excellent qualities. This includes engaging in gentle, not aggressive or overbearing, speech which promotes harmonious relationships. When someone generally treats one well, but on occasion acts inappropriately by speaking harshly and so on, it is wrong to retaliate with sarcasm or abuse. Rather, one should listen to the person's criticism and respond to it in a gentle fashion. Especially if one is abused or harmed in some other way by an enemy, it is important not to retaliate, but to be forebearing. By so doing, one may find over time that the enemy becomes one's friend.

One should show respect to those who have helped one in times of need, and to teachers and older relatives. This was the normal behavior in Tibet, but that tradition has deteriorated there as a result of the Chinese Communist occupation. Generally speaking, it is important to speak and act in accordance with the customs of the country where one is living and to behave harmoniously with one's friends and companions.

Whatever one's livelihood, it should be conducted conscientiously, and one should not be excessively parsimonious. A Tibetan aphorism states: "If you are living in a house in which even the rafters are made of solid gold, do not be stingy even with water. If there is a real need, shave the gold off your rafters."

Spiritual Conduct

Regardless of one's occupation—whether it is farming, business, or factory work—and regardless of how hard one works, if one engages in no spiritual practice, then all one's hard work simply acts as a source of suffering in future lives. Therefore, in order to avoid suffering and bring about genuine happiness one should engage in spiritual practice. We can see this for ourselves. There are many rich individuals who devote a tremendous amount of time to work, and yet they find no real happiness and their minds are fraught with anxiety. In the meantime, they are simply sowing seeds for miserable rebirths such as *pretas* or denizens of hell realms. Even if one wishes eventually to engage in spiritual practice, but puts it off while pursuing other priorities of accumulating wealth and so on, the only time left over for spiritual practice will come when one's body is resting in a casket.

As mentioned earlier, the ten nonvirtuous activities especially to be avoided are the three physical acts of killing, sexual misconduct, and stealing; the four verbal acts are lying, slander, abuse, and idle gossip; and the three mental nonvirtues are avarice, malice, and holding false views. To aid one's spiritual practice, it is very helpful to devote oneself to a spiritual mentor in whom one has faith. One should not simply follow someone who is famous, but rather a person with excellent qualities with whom one has a genuine relationship. Actually, many famous spiritual teachers do not lead exemplary lives, so one should closely examine a person whom one is considering as a spiritual mentor to see whether he or she truly has excellent qualities. If one establishes this relationship with a mentor, one should seek guidance and follow whatever spiritual counsel one receives. In a proper relationship one can receive great blessings from such a teacher. It is not possible, though, for the teacher simply to impart his or her realization to the student. The Buddha himself said that even he was not able to remove others' sufferings directly, nor could he directly impart to others his own realization. The principal way a teacher serves others is to impart spiritual guidance, which gradually brings benefit if the student puts it into practice. I have heard people in the West claim to actually transmit their realizations to other people, but I am very skeptical of such claims.

A particularly helpful type of spiritual practice is to cultivate the four immeasurables of loving-kindness, compassion, empathetic joy, and equanimity. When one witnesses other people in physical or mental suffering due to illness, poverty or any other adversity, one should help them out in any way possible. I find that such altruistic service is laudably common in the modern West, perhaps even more so than in some Buddhist societies. One should cherish the lives of all other beings as one does one's own, for all sentient beings including insects, like oneself, wish to avoid suffering and find happiness. Thus, one should avoid harming them, including those animals that are regarded simply as food, and help them in their pursuit of happiness.

In addition, one should cultivate the six perfections, which provide the framework for the *bodhisattva* way of life, namely: the perfection of generosity, discipline, patience, zeal, meditation, and wisdom. Among the many types of generosity, the most important is the gift of protection. If one can protect another sentient being whose life or well-being is in danger, this is the greatest of gifts. In this case, even lying to protect others is acceptable. For example, imagine the case of a hunter tracking a deer. If the deer runs by you and is followed by the hunter who asks you where the deer ran to, it is quite appropriate to say you did not see it, even if you saw it perfectly well. Or, if you saw the deer run up the mountain, you could well reply that you saw it run down the mountain.

The second perfection of ethical discipline refers especially to avoiding the ten nonvirtues of the body, speech, and mind. The perfection of patience is extremely important, for if one lacks patience, then hatred, jealousy, and pride are bound to arise in one's mind-stream and dominate one's behavior. Even if one is being beaten, by cultivating patience one does not retaliate. As the eighth-century Indian *bodhisattva* Śāntideva states in his classic treatise *A Guide to the Bodhisattva Way of Life,* "There

---

74. *A Guide to the Bodhisattva Way of Life,* trans. by Vesna A. Wallace & B. Alan Wallace (Ithaca: Snow Lion, 1997), VI: 2.

is no vice like hatred, and there is no austerity like patience."[74] In another verse he declares, "Where would there be leather enough to cover the entire world? With just the leather of my sandals, it is as if the whole earth were covered. Likewise, I am unable to restrain external phenomena, but I shall restrain my own mind. What need is there to restrain anything else?"[75] There is no end to the thorns of adversities and problems that arise in the course of life, so it is futile to try to transform the entire environment and all the people in it so that nothing is disagreeable. Rather, one should simply cultivate patience and forebearance, like cladding one's own feet in leather instead of trying to cover the whole earth with leather. When anger or hatred arises, one is usually focused on the object that has aroused one's aggression. But if one can attend to the anger itself and identify its nature as it is arising, without acting on it, that is excellent. If one can identify any affliction of the mind when it arises, it can gradually become attenuated. The other perfections of patience, zeal, meditation, and wisdom are discussed in many works on Buddhism, so I shall not elaborate on them at this time.

Seasonal Behavior

Seasonal behavior is explained in terms of the six seasons of the year, namely early winter, late winter, spring, summer, monsoon, and autumn, each of which lasts two months. The smallest division of experiential time is the duration of a single pulse of consciousness. The duration of 120 of such pulses is one instant. Sixty instants make one moment, thirty such moments make one period, and thirty such periods make one day and night.[76] A month consists of thirty days, a season consists of two months, and a year consists of six seasons.

The summer and winter solstices fall in the middle of the summer and winter, during the fifth and eleventh Tibetan months. Therefore, for three seasons the sun moves to the south, and for three it moves to the north. The spring and autumn equinoxes come halfway through each cycle of three seasons, during the second and eighth Tibetan months. As

---

75. Ibid., V: 13-14.

76. Translator's note: This mode of reckoning implies that the duration of a single moment of consciousness is roughly 0.01 seconds, the duration of one instant is 1.6 seconds, one moment is 96 seconds, and one period lasts 48 minutes.

the sun begins moving to the north, from the twelfth Tibetan month, the power of the sun and the air element gradually increase, with their sharp, hot, and coarse qualities, while simultaneously diminishing the qualities of the moon and the earth element.

During that time, strong hot, astringent, and bitter flavors diminish the strength and vigor of human beings. Human strength increases gradually as the strength of the moon increases and the sun declines. At that time the environment is especially imbued with sour, salty, and sweet flavors. Human strength is at its peak during the winter, at its lowest during the summer and monsoon, and medium during the autumn and spring.

As for wholesome behavior pertaining to the six seasons, due to the cold of early winter, the pores are constricted and the power of the digestive warmth increases, like a fire aroused by the wind. If one eats too little food, this will decrease the bodily constituents, so one should consume adequate amounts of food, especially those that are sweet, sour, and salty. Due to the long nights during this season, one tends to feel hungry and the bodily constituents may deteriorate. To counteract this, one should apply sesame oil on the body, consume meat soup and oily foods, wear warm clothing, and live in a warm, well-insulated lodging. Late winter is extremely cold, so the same behavioral advice applies to that season.

Phlegm disorders accumulated during the winter are aroused in the spring due to the increased warmth of the sun and the decrease of the digestive warmth. To counteract such disorders that may arise during this season, one should eat foods having bitter, hot, and astringent tastes. One should also consume aged grain, the meat of animals that live on dry land, honey, hot boiled water, ginger decoctions, and coarse-powered foods and beverages. Phlegm imbalances are also remedied by vigorous walking and rubbing pea flour on the body, and it may also be helpful to sit in fragrant and shady groves.

During the summer the great heat of the sun's rays consumes one's strength, so one should avoid foods having salty, hot, and sour tastes, strenuous activities, and sitting in the sun. One also should consume sweet, light, oily, and cooling powered foods and beverages, take baths with cool water, drink alcoholic beverages diluted with water, wear light clothing, and sit in cool and fragrant dwellings. It may also be helpful to expose oneself to moist wind and cool breezes, and to sit in the shade of the trees.

During the monsoon, clouds gather in the sky and rain moistens the land. Consequently, wind, cold, vapor from the earth, and turbid and contaminated water impair the digestive warmth. To increase the digestive warmth, one should eat foods that are sweet, sour, salty, light, and warming, as well as oily-powered foods and beverages. One should also drink alcoholic beverages made from grain and sit in elevated places to avoid the coolness of the ground.

In the autumn, the sun's rays striking the body arouse bile disorders, which accumulate during the monsoon. To pacify such disorders one should eat sweet, bitter, and astringent food, wear clothing scented with camphor and sandalwood, and sit inside on a floor sprinkled with water.

In summary, one should take warming foods and beverages during the monsoon and winter, coarse food and drink in the spring, and cooling food and drink in the summer and autumn. One should emphasize sweet, sour, and salty foods during the monsoon and winter; bitter, hot, and astringent foods during the spring; sweet foods in the summer; and sweet, bitter, and astringent foods during the autumn. Purgatives, emetics, and suppositories are recommended during the autumn, spring, and monsoon respectively. One should analyze carefully whether the treatments given are inadequate, excessive or wrong.[77]

Occasional Behavior

The Tibetan medical discussion of occasional behavior addresses thirteen topics: (1) hunger, (2) thirst, (3) vomiting, (4) sneezing, (5) yawning, (6) breathing, (7) sleeping, (8) sputum, (9) saliva, (10) intestinal gas, (11) defecation, (12) urination, and (13) ejaculation.

(1) The simple advice regarding hunger is that when one feels hungry, one should eat. If one makes a habit of going without food even when hungry, this leads to a weakening of the body, dizziness, and dysphagia (and anorexia). If one is involuntarily deprived of food for some time, it is important initially that one does not eat very rich or difficult to digest food, such as meat; rather, one should eat easily digestible foods such as rice gruel or cooked barley flour, which is the staple diet of Tibet, meat

---

77. Translator's note: For further descriptions of seasonal behavior see Dr. Yeshi Donden, *Health Through Balance*, ed. & trans. by Jeffrey Hopkins (Ithaca: Snow Lion, 1986), pp. 144-148, and the *Encyclopedia of Tibetan Medicine*, Vol. III, Ch. 14.

broth, and butter. This is the way to restore one's health and appetite.

(2) Likewise, when one is thirsty, it is important to drink water, for when the body is deprived of liquid, this leads to dizziness, stomach disorders, an imbalance of the "heart wind," attentional instability, and memory loss. If one involuntarily becomes dehydrated, one should initially splash water on the face, then begin drinking in small sips. In the meantime, one should stay in a cool location and not engage in strenuous activity. Since dehydration leads to wind disorders, it can be helpful to drink something with a very low alcohol content, such as diluted beer.

In all the towns and cities of traditional Tibet, if one was invited as a guest to any household, one would always be given food, regardless of whether one was a Tibetan, a Westerner, or a Chinese. When beggars came to one's door for alms, people who did not want to give them their finest beer would give them watered down beer and a little bit of parched barley meal. But to their close friends or people whom they wanted to honor they would offer full-strength beer. Sometimes when beggars would come to a household hoping for the good brew and receive a watered down beer instead, they would comment, "We came with high hopes, but they just gave us the watered down stuff." That being said, if someone comes to you who is dehydrated, you may give them weak beer and not feel guilty about it.

(3) If one feels the urge to vomit, one should definitely allow oneself to do so, for if one habitually restrains oneself from vomiting, this can give rise to respiratory problems, swelling of the chest and face, erysipelas, chronic lesions on the skin, discomfort in the eyes, excessive sputum, coughing up of sputum, and increased vulnerability to contagious illnesses such as colds and flu. If one has been prone to vomiting but has habitually restrained oneself, to restore one's health one should fast, and drink a tea made from powdered red sandalwood, eaglewood (or aloewood), costus root, and the root of a flower called in Tibetan *pukar* (*spu dkar*). This infusion should be drunk by the spoonful, holding each spoonful in the mouth before swallowing it.

(4) When inclined to sneeze it is important not to restrain oneself. Inhibiting sneezing can lead to unclarity of vision and hearing, headaches, stiffness in the back of the neck, strain on the muscles around the mouth, and wind disorders. To counteract such problems created by inhibiting sneezing, one should inhale incense made from sandalwood and eaglewood (or aloewood). In Tibet such incense would be poured over embers glow-

ing in a large pot, and people would inhale the smoke through a pipe.

(5) Likewise, one should not prevent oneself from yawning. The imbalances arising from inhibiting yawning can be counteracted by inhaling the above incense and by taking medicine for a wind disorder.

(6) Due to thinking too much or experiencing intense fear or suffering, one's respiration may be inhibited, such that one feels a need to breathe deeply or sigh. Even in times of powerful grief, anxiety, or fear it is important not to let these emotions interfere with one's breathing. If one's respiration is inhibited by these intense emotions, this can give rise to disorders in the heart and to tumors that originate from a wind imbalance. Improper breathing can also lead to mental imbalances, including insanity and catatonia. When such disorders arise, one should take medication to treat wind imbalances, avoid stress, and take one's mind away from the source of fear or sorrow, for example by engaging in warm conversation with a friendly, cheerful person.

In the Tibetan tradition such mental afflictions are viewed and treated differently than in Western psychology and psychiatry. For instance, in some cases mental imbalances are attributed to spirits, and these are treated with a combination of medication for wind imbalances and advice concerning the person's diet and conduct pertaining to the body, speech, and mind. Mental afflictions may be related to wind, bile, or phlegm. Different types of environment, diet, and conduct are prescribed for a mental imbalance due to a wind disorder, a bile disorder, and a phlegm disorder. Thus, mental imbalances are closely related to a person's humoral constitution, and this must be identified by a fully qualified Tibetan physician so that each case can be treated individually. That is part of the standard Tibetan medical training, not a separate specialty.

(7) It is important not to become sleep deprived. If one makes a habit of sleeping too little, this can lead to various disorders having the following symptoms: yawning, lethargy, heaviness of the head, lack of mental clarity, and indigestion. To remedy such problems, one should first drink mutton broth and fresh beer. In Tibet people would often drink barley beer only three days old. Aged beer, in contrast, tends to be very potent, and drinking it can lead to rowdy, aggressive behavior. In addition, one should massage the body with a mixture of sesame oil and melted butter.

To counteract sleep deprivation, in the wintertime, when the nights are long, one may sleep at any time, day or night. In the spring or summertime, when the nights are much shorter, if one sleeps too little one night, it is important to catch up on one's sleep the very next day.

(8) If one coughs up sputum, it is healthy to spit it out and not swallow it. If one does constantly swallow one's sputum, it will increase and can lead to respiratory problems, such as asthma, weight loss, hiccups, heart disorders, and loss of appetite. To counteract such problems, one should drink an infusion of ginger, pepper, and raw sugar.

(9) If excessive saliva accumulates in the mouth, one may either spit it out or swallow it, but one should not retain it in the mouth, for this can lead to disorders in the heart and the head, runny nose, dizziness, and loss of appetite. The remedy for such problems is to drink beer, sleep, and engage in pleasant conversation with agreeable people.

(10) Intestinal gas should be let out in an appropriate place, for restraining it leads to dryness of the feces and constipation, abdominal bloating, tumors, unclear vision, decrease of digestive warmth, and heart disorders. The remedies for such problems are the same as those for problems due to inhibiting defecation, which is the next topic.

(11) If one inhibits defecation, this can lead to an inversion of the digestive process resulting in foul breath and vomiting, brain disorders, spasms in the calves, and increased vulnerability to the common cold. There are two types of treatment for problems resulting from blocked intestinal gas or feces. The first of these is a kind of mild laxative inserted into the sphincter, while the patient lies on his back with his feet up, and it is held inside for as long as one or two hours. During that time, at least for half an hour or so, the patient lying on his back claps his feet together. This is very helpful for wind disorders. After an hour or two, one will defecate quite easily.

The second treatment is a fast-acting purgative enema that induces a bowel movement within minutes. The proper quantity of this medication, ranging from one to three cups, depends on the health of the patient. Generally speaking, a mild laxative is helpful for wind disorders; a strong purgative can be useful for bile disorders; and an emetic can be helpful for phlegm disorders.

(12) Inhibiting urination can lead to the formation of stones in the urinary bladder, discomfort in the urinary tract and the inside of the thigh, and disorders of the descending wind. A mild purgative enema is the best treatment for such problems. Immersion in hot springs or mineral baths, massage with sesame oil, and wrapping one's waist with a wolf

or lynx hide or sitting on such a hide can also be helpful.

This final remedy traces back to the folk medicine of ancient Tibet. In Tibet there has been a lot of discussion concerning whether *The Four Tantras* are really the teachings of the Buddha, whether they were originally *termas* ("hidden treasures"), or whether they were drawn from the Bön religion, which is indigenous to Tibet. I believe the essential nature of these treatises is that of the words of the Buddha himself. These treatises can be traced back to the time of Padmasambhava and Vairocana in the eighth century.[78] For over five thousand years, *The Four Tantras* were preserved in Tibet solely as an oral lineage (tracing back to the Sovereign Healer himself), but during the reign of King Trisong Detsen, a *ḍākinī*[79] appeared in a dream to Yuthok Yönten Gönpo and told him to go to India to receive teachings from the renowned doctors Biji Gadjé and Bihla Gadzey, both of whom had achieved the *siddhi*[80] of immortality. While Yuthok Yönten Gönpo was on his way to India, he encountered Vairocana, who was returning from India, where he had been studying with the Indian Paṇḍit Candradeva. Vairocana told him that he did not need to go to India, for Paṇḍit Candradeva had given him a copy of *The Four Tantras* with the instructions to give them to Yuthok Yönten Gönpo. But Yuthok Yönten Gönpo continued on to India anyway and achieved his goal of meeting with Biji Gadjé and Bihla Gadzey and receiving medical instruction from them. In addition, he had a vision of Nāgārjuna, who had passed away years earlier.

Yuthok Yönten Gönpo then made his way back to Tibet, and on his return journey he met two translators from Samye Monastery, Kawa Betse and Chokrong Lü Gyaltsen, who were on their way to India to invite the Buddhist master Vimalamitra to Tibet. Yuthok Yönten Gönpo asked them what had become of *The Four Tantras* that Vairocana had brought with him to Tibet. They replied that Vairocana had offered them to King

---

78. Padmasambhava was the founder of the Nyingma order of Tibetan Buddhism, and Vairocana was the first of the great translators also of that same school.

79. Translator's note: Tib. *mkha' 'gro ma*. A highly realized female *bodhisattva* who manifests in the world in order to serve sentient beings. Literally, the term means a female "sky-goer," referring to the fact that such beings course in the expanse of the absolute nature of reality.

80. Translator's note: Tib. *dngos sgrub*. A paranormal ability.

Trisong Detsen, who had then concealed them as a *terma* in a hollow pillar at Samye. Since these texts were temporarily unavailable, he returned to India, where he received complete instructions on *The Four Tantras*, as well as the texts themselves, from Paṇḍit Candradeva. When he brought these back to Tibet, this allowed for a confluence of oral and textual transmissions of these *tantras*. Many years later, the contemplative Drapa Ngönshey revealed the *terma* of *The Four Tantras* hidden in the hollow pillar at Samye. It turned out that the meaning of the different versions of *The Four Tantras* that had been concealed at Samye and that had been brought from India by Yuthok Yönten Gönpo was essentially the same.

In addition to the medical teachings coming to Tibet from India, the Tibetans had acquired a great deal of their own indigenous medical knowledge, which they then integrated with the medical teachings they received from India. Tibetan medicine today consists of an integration of these strands of medical knowledge.

(13) The Tibetan term translated in these lectures as "regenerative substances" (*khu ba*) sometimes refers to both the ovum and the semen, but in this case it refers to the semen alone. If one habitually blocks the flow of semen, this can lead to the involuntary loss, or leakage, or semen, blockage of the tip of the penis, obstruction of urination, the formation of stones in the kidneys and the urinary bladder, or one may become impotent.

In the Buddhist tradition, a boy must be at least eight years old before taking the novice precepts of a monk, and one must be at least twenty before taking full ordination. Especially once one becomes fully ordained, one must be strictly celibate, so one never voluntarily emits semen. If one takes the vow of chastity before the age of twenty, an adolescent male may experience a sex change. In this case, the male genitals dry up and diminish in size until they take on the characteristics of a woman's genitals. One also grows breasts, and the seminal vesicle is drawn inside the abdomen instead of being located by the testicles. Such a sex change can happen during adolescence or even as late as eighteen years of age, and this is the reason why males are not allowed to take full ordination until that age. In the West this does not appear to be a problem, because many people are already sexually active by the age of fifteen or younger, and once one is sexually active one will not experience such an involuntary sex change. In Tibet there were many cases of sex changes from male to female, but it is extremely difficult, if not impossible, to change from female to male. The remedies for problems cited earlier due to the blockage of semen are to drink milk and good beer.

It is important not to block any of the above functions, especially not forcefully. It is also important not to defecate or urinate very forcefully, for this can lead to various diseases by creating wind imbalances.

Questions and Responses

QUESTION: In one of your personal anecdotes you mentioned that you advised a woman patient to go to a *lama* for divination concerning the hospital she should go to. What are your criteria for deciding to send a patient to a *lama* for a divination, instead of determining by yourself alone how to treat the patient medically?

RESPONSE: Such a question is quite natural in the West, because there is no tradition of Western doctors advising their patients to consult a clergyman for a divination. But this was a common custom in traditional Tibet. If someone in a village were to fall ill, those close to him would commonly first consult a trusted *lama* to help with the choice of a doctor. Tibetan doctors have somewhat different ways of diagnosing illnesses and preparing medicines. When a *lama* performs a divination, he is usually consulting a mundane (unenlightened) *deva,* or god. This is still done nowadays in Dharmsala, India, where there is a variety of doctors from which to choose. One may go to a Tibetan doctor, a Western-trained Indian doctor, or an Āyurvedic doctor. While performing a divination, a *lama* might also inquire into the kind of medicine the person should take and the hospital he should go to. If an illness originated primarily from a demonic influence, the *lama* might not send the patient to a doctor at all, but rather send him to a tantric adept, who would use paranormal methods for alleviating the illness. There are many invisible influences that can cause diseases, and they may be remedied by methods that are also invisible. When a Tibetan doctor needs to make a decision about a patient, but lacks sufficient medical information to do so, he will likely encourage the patient to request a *lama* for a divination.

I previously mentioned that one of the characteristics of a superior physician is clairvoyance, enabling one to recognize the exact nature of a disease without being told or performing a diagnosis. Such clairvoyance can be achieved by certain types of Buddhist meditation, which were part of traditional Tibetan medical training. A supreme physician is a *buddha*, who has unimpeded clairvoyance. Many doctors in the history of Tibetan medicine are regarded as emanations of the *buddhas*. Those are the best physicians, and there have been many other physicians and *lamas* who have accomplished various types of extrasensory perception, even though they were not perfectly enlightened. When such a *lama* was asked to perform a divination, he might go through the motions of doing this ritual, but in fact he could see what needed to be done by means of his extrasensory perception.

The Explanatory Tantra says that a well-trained physician should be like a person who has ascended a mountain and can see unimpededly in all directions. Such knowledge comes from thorough training. If one becomes a total expert in the principal forms of diagnosis—urine and pulse diagnosis—one's intuition and senses can become so refined that it is as if one had extrasensory perception. Moreover, in the full, traditional training in Tibetan medicine, one studies various ritual practices, including *mantra* recitation, pertaining to the Medicine Buddha. Secondly, one learns how to prescribe medical treatments; and thirdly, one trains in meditative concentration (*samādhi*). If one is accomplished in all three of these approaches, extrasensory perception could also be used in making one's diagnosis.

Although I have briefly mentioned urine analysis, I have said very little about pulse diagnosis, which is an elaborate topic in Tibetan medicine. In this context, there is the whole branch of diagnosis pertaining to the "seven wondrous pulses."[81] A physician who has learned how to identify these pulses may, for example, accurately diagnose an ill husband, who is bedridden and unable to visit the doctor, by examining the pulse of his wife, or vice versa. He may examine a mother's pulse and thereby diagnose her child. Such cross-diagnosis can also be practiced among brothers and sisters. I will not try to explain the underlying theory for this practice, though, for it would be virtually impossible for modern Westerners to practice this. As the late, eminent Tibetan contemplative

---

81. Translator's note: In the *Bod rgya tshig mdzod chen mo* (Chengdu: Mi rigs dpe skrun khang, 1984, p. 666) these are listed as: (1) *khyim phyva*, (2) *mgron phyva*, (3) *dgra phyva*, (4) *grogs phyva*, (5) *gdon phyva*, (6) *me chu go ldog*, and (7) *bu rtsa*.

Kalu Rinpoche commented, "In these days there is more and more talk and less and less practice." I could say a good deal about these wondrous pulses, but it would lead only to more talk, taking us away from more practical matters.

QUESTION: In certain tantric practices one must retain the semen. Does such practice make one prone to the kinds of problems mentioned earlier?

RESPONSE: There are indeed tantric practices in which the semen is not to be emitted, but in such advanced practices, one learns to emit and then retract the semen. This can be done only with a high degree of mastery over one's vital energies, and such practice does not make one ill. In this type of tantric practice, women do not retain any regenerative substance. Rather, if they are generating themselves as the male deity Kālacakra, they dissolve their identity as a woman and imagine themselves in the form of the male deity. This visualization should be so vivid and clear that one can mentally see it as vividly as if one were looking in a mirror. There are other tantric practices, such as Vajrayoginī, in which the principal deity is female, and in such practices both men and women imagine themselves in the form of the female deity. These are very difficult techniques and are not to be practiced without preparation. At the very least, one must be well versed in the nature of *karma*, of actions and their long-term consequences, and understand the ground, path, and fruition of tantric practice.

Chapter Sixteen
The Potencies of Tastes

To understand the rationale behind the Tibetan medical views concerning a wholesome diet, one should learn the specific potencies of tastes. The Tibetan medical explanation concerning tastes addresses five topics: (1) the bases for the six tastes, (2) the classification of tastes, (3) the essential natures of tastes, (4) the therapeutic efficacies of tastes, and (5) the functions of tastes.

(1) The basis for the six tastes is the five elements. Among the elements, earth acts as the fundamental basis; water provides fluidity and moisture; fire provides warmth and allows for maturation; air creates growth; and space provides the dimension in which growth can take place.

(2) The classification of tastes includes bitter, astringent, sweet, sour, salty, and hot tastes. In any given substance, although all five elements are present, if earth and water are dominant, this gives rise to a sweet taste; if earth and fire elements are dominant, this gives rise to a sour taste; if water and fire are dominant, this gives rise to a salty taste; if water and air are dominant, this gives rise to a bitter taste; if fire and air are dominant, this gives rise to a hot taste; and if earth and air are dominant, this gives rise to an astringent taste.

(3) As for the essential natures of the six tastes, when one experiences a sweet taste, desire arises and one wants to eat more. When one experiences a sour taste, it makes the teeth ache, contorts the face, and causes salivation. When one experiences a salty taste, it makes the tongue burn

and also causes salivation. When one experiences a bitter taste, it cleanses odors in the mouth and counteracts hiccups. When one experiences a hot taste, the mouth and tongue burn, and tears come to the eyes. When one experiences an astringent taste, it cleaves to the palate, it is rough, and does not leave much of a taste.

(4) Among the potencies of each of the elements, earth is heavy, stable, dull, smooth, oily, and dry; and this element counteracts wind disorders, which are closely associated with the air element, both of which are light, motile, cold, and subtle. The lightness of the air element and the wind humor is counteracted by the heaviness of the earth, and the motility of the air is counteracted by the stability of the earth element. Water is fluid, cool, heavy, dull, oily, and supple, and its potencies counteract bile disorders. Bile is sharp, hot, light, and oily, and its sharp and hot qualities are especially counteracted by the cool and dull potencies of water. Fire is hot, sharp, dry, rough, light, oily,[82] and motile, and its potencies counteract imbalances of phlegm, which is heavy, dull, smooth, oily, and sticky. Air is light, motile, cold, rough, dry (opposite of oily), and subtle, and its potencies counteract disorders of both phlegm and bile. The element of space pervades the other four elements. All the potencies of each of the elements and their therapeutic efficacies need to be taken into account by a Tibetan physician when preparing medical compounds.

(5) The earth element has the function of giving substance, or firmness, to the various constituents of the body, and it counteracts wind disorders. The function of the water element is to moisten the various constituents of the body and make them supple; and together with the earth element, the water element holds the body together. Water counteracts bile disorders, which are more or less equivalent to heat disorders. Fire brings warmth to the body, assists in the digestion of food and drink, brings color to the body, clears one's complexion, and counteracts phlegm disorders. The air element is the basis of tactile sensations and is responsible for all types of bodily movements, acting to circulate fluids such as

---

82. The rationale for the oily potency of fire is that a substance after it is burned tends to have an oily quality. In reality, all the potencies of the elements are relational, rather than intrinsic to the elements themselves. This is because, according to Madhyamaka philosophy, which is generally considered the pinnacle of Buddhist thought, no phenomenon exists in and of itself; everything consists of dependently related events, rather than independent substances.

the nutriment, lymph, and blood throughout the body. It counteracts both phlegm and bile disorders. The space element includes and pervades the other four elements, and is the basis for the audial faculty. Moreover, all cavities within the body are of the nature of space.

All types of medication, the six tastes, and the body itself all originate from the five elements. As one eats food and drink having any of the six tastes, they contribute to the corresponding elements within the body. Moreover, when one's diet and behavior are unhealthy, this leads to an excess, deficiency, or disturbance of the humors. There are no medical ingredients that do not originate from and include the earth element. As stated in *The Final Tantra,* all emetics and other medications designed to treat phlegm disorders are dominant in the fire and air elements, for these two elements together have the nature of moving upwards. Laxatives and medicines to induce urination are dominant in the earth and water elements. Most sweet foods and drinks have a heavy quality due to the dominance of earth and water. Medical compounds made from raw, sweet ingredients tend to have a laxative quality, but they may induce harmful side-effects. There is nothing on the planet that cannot be used in medicine.

Among the six tastes, a hot taste overpowers an astringent taste; bitter overpowers hot; salty overpowers bitter; sour overpowers salty; and sweet overpowers sour. The subtle interactions among these various tastes are very complex and difficult to understand. To give a few examples, if a medical ingredient dominant in the earth element (which is heavy) is combined with an ingredient dominant in water (which is also heavy), the compound would have an exceptionally heavy potency. If the firm potency of earth interacts with the gentle potency of water, the firmness of earth overpowers the gentle potency of water. Between the oiliness of earth and the fluidity of water, fluidity dominates over oiliness. When the rough and light potencies of fire interact, they tend to neutralize each other. One of the potencies of earth is the quality of smoothness. One of the qualities of fire is roughness. Between the smooth potency of earth and the rough potency of fire, the rough potency dominates over the smooth potency. Among the complex interactions of the potencies of the various tastes, sometimes one potency enhances another, and sometimes one neutralizes the other.

To give some further background on the Tibetan medical heritage, the personal physician of the Fifth Dalai Lama was named Darmo Lobzang Chödrak, who was born in the Darmo region of southern Tibet.[83] This doctor, who was held in very high regard by the Fifth Dalai Lama, combined the Zurpa and Jangpa medical lineages, each of which has its own interpretation of *The Four Tantras,* and founded the Chakpori Medical College. At this time another prominent physician named Sönam Wangden, who was a good friend of Lobzang Chödrak, lived in a large monastery in the south of Tibet, where he taught medicine. Sometimes Sönam Wangden would go to Gohara in eastern India on business, and he knew the route well from southern Tibet to eastern India.

At that time, the Fifth Dalai Lama, unbeknownst to Sangye Gyatso (who was to become Regent of Tibet following the Dalai Lama's death), secretly gave Lobzang Chödrak gold with instructions to accompany Sönam Wangden to Gohara to learn what he could from the Indian Buddhists who had fled there to escape the oppression of the Moslems, who had conquered India. When they arrived in Gohara, they met with a number of learned physicians from whom Lobzang Chödrak learned a great deal about certain oral lineages and other practical medical teachings. He took notes on what he learned and returned to Lhasa, where he planned to publish his findings. However, the Fifth Dalai Lama passed away before he could bring his plans to fruition.

When the Regent Sangye Gyatso was in power, many disturbances arose in Tibet, which forced Lobzang Chödrak into exile. He was invited by the great Buddhist scholar Jamyang Shäpa, who had trained in Gomang College of Drepung Monastic University in Central Tibet, to come to his home monastery, Tashi Kyil in the Amdo region of Eastern Tibet. Both Jamyang Shäpa and his next incarnation, Jigmé Wangpo, revered him, and he founded a medical school at Tashi Kyil. Lobzang Chödrak composed four volumes on Tibetan medicine, entitled *The Hundred Works of Darmo,* which contained much new information, and these were published in Kumbum and in Degé. He then spent a good deal of time in Amdo near the border of Mongolia, and the Mongolians preserved many of his treatises. Unless the wood-blocks for these texts were destroyed, I

---

83. When I was a young boy, some people believed I was an incarnation of this doctor, but I have no recollection of such a previous life (I can't even remember what I had for breakfast yesterday!).

believe they are still extant both at Kumbum and Degé.

Once tastes have been processed by the decomposing phlegm, the digestive bile, and the fire-accompanying wind, sweet and salty tastes become sweet; sour tastes remain sour; and bitter, hot, and astringent tastes become bitter. Among the humoral disorders, wind and bile disorders are dispelled by a post-digestive sweet taste; phlegm and wind disorders are dispelled by a post-digestive sour taste; and phlegm and bile disorders are dispelled by a post-digestive bitter taste. That is why it is said that two types of disorders are dispelled by a single taste. Whatever qualities a medicine may have, they are attributed to the tastes of its ingredients. Medicines affect the body by way of the elements of which they are composed, and each of the elements is associated with specific tastes, as explained before. The post-digestive potencies of the various tastes supersede their initial potencies, but both types of potencies have an impact on the body. To give a general example, a sweet taste remains sweet after digestion, and both the initial and post-digestive sweet tastes have a heavy quality, so both counteract wind disorders, which are light by nature.

The Ancestral Oral Tradition, a four-volume commentary on *The Four Tantras* according to the Zurpa lineage, states that the explanation of post-digestive tastes refers to the potencies of the tastes after they have been entirely processed by the phlegm, bile, and wind. However, these post-digestive tastes especially result from the interaction of the initial tastes with the decomposing phlegm. There is much diverse information in Tibetan medical literature, which extends far beyond *The Four Tantras.* Even among the versions of *The Four Tantras,* there are *termas* (concealed treasures), *kamas* (canonical versions of *The Four Tantras* translated from Sanskrit into Tibetan), and oral lineages transmitted over the generations from teacher to disciple. Many of those oral lineages actually predate the first written appearance of *The Four Tantras* in Tibet.

In ancient Tibet many medical ingredients had been identified and used in making medical compounds. To illustrate the antiquity of this medical tradition, there is an herbal compound called Choka Chejor 25 that has twenty-five ingredients and traces back further than the reign of the Tibetan kings, that is, more than 2,123 years ago. A *choka* is similar to a cuckoo. In ancient times, Tibetans would seek out the *choka's* nest and paint red dye on the eggs. When the mother bird returned to her eggs, she presumably thought they had been broken, so she went off to gather various herbs and applied them to the eggs to mend them. The Tibetans then observed the herbs she gathered and from this identified those that would heal wounds.

Tibetans also observed another bird called a *ja-ngar*, similar to the wild turkey in North America. Once its chicks had hatched and were walking around, Tibetans would catch the chicks and smear blood on them. The mother bird, thinking they had been wounded, would gather herbs and apply them to her chicks. Once again, the Tibetans would observe the herbs she brought. They would also apply this technique to monkeys, smearing them with the blood of another animal, and then watching what types of plants they would apply to bind and heal the "wounds" of their kin. Another method tracing back more than two thousand years was to smear charcoal on an animal, such as a baby rabbit, to make its parents think it was injured. Then these early Tibetans would watch to see what types of herbs the parents would bring to heal their ostensibly sick young. By engaging in such naturalistic research, Tibetans identified twenty-five different plant substances that could be used for various types of wounds and other disorders.

On another occasion, a king saw his wife kill a frog, and he became concerned at this, for according to Tibetan tradition, frogs are sometimes associated with the *nāgas*, which are responsible for various types of skin disorders. After some time, the king became afflicted with leprosy. He then removed himself from his whole family and went to a charnel ground, where he remained in isolation. People left food for him at designated drop-points. He quarantined himself in this way, because he knew that leprosy was contagious; and there came to be a general tradition in Tibet prohibiting people from traveling from regions where there were epidemics of infectious diseases. The ancient Tibetans were not stupid or ignorant, but people gradually came to ignore what had been learned in earlier times; so some of the earlier knowledge was lost.

Chapter Seventeen
Wholesome Diet

In the medical *tantras* three chapters are devoted to the topic of a wholesome diet, but here I shall address only the third of those chapters, which explains the amounts of food that are most conducive to good health.[84] Each person must judge for himself how much is appropriate to eat. In this regard one must take into account the heaviness or lightness of the food in relationship to the strength of one's own digestive warmth. One may eat as much light food as one wishes, but it is important to eat heavy or rich food only in moderate quantities; for light foods are easy to digest, whereas heavy foods are difficult to digest. Moreover, if one chooses to drink any kind of alcoholic beverage, it is important to do so in moderation and not to the point of intoxication.

One's dietary habits have a great bearing on one's longevity. The classical texts explain this point with a metaphor: eating is like sowing a field with grain. Likewise, with a healthy diet, one's digestive warmth is maintained, and this leads to a "harvest" of good health. An unhealthy diet, on the other hand, impairs one's digestive warmth, which then damages one's health. Therefore, if one eats healthy amounts of heavy and light

---

84. Translator's note: Dr. Dhonden discussed the qualities of different kinds of food in *Health Through Balance* in chapters 12 & 13. A more elaborate explanation is found in the *Encyclopedia of Tibetan Medicine*, Vaidya Bhagwan Dash (Delhi: Sri Satguru Publications, 1994), Vol. III, Chs. 16-18. There the topic of quantity of food intake is discussed in Ch. 18.

foods in accordance with one's digestive ability, this increases the strength of the body, enhances one's complexion, and gives rise to long life. This advice pertains to one's diet throughout all seasons, though it is also true that during the summer, when the days are long, one should eat light food; and in the winter, one may eat heavier, or richer, food.

On the other hand, there are disadvantages to eating too little: one's physical strength wanes, one's complexion deteriorates, and this leads to all manner of wind disorders. Moreover, if one chooses food purely for its taste, eating many sweets, for example, this impairs one's digestive warmth, which leads to phlegm disorders. If one does not know the appropriate amounts of food and drink to take, one is bound to fall to one extreme or another. Generally speaking, too little food and drink leads to wind disorders, sadness, depression, and other mental afflictions; while excessive food leads to phlegm disorders, which originate in the stomach, then spread elsewhere. In short, one should choose one's food, not simply on the basis of how it tastes, but rather on the basis of how well one can digest it.

As for the appropriate proportions of food and drink in a single meal, according to the classic Tibetan tradition, one-fourth of the volume of the stomach should be filled with solid food, one-half should be filled with fluids, and one-fourth should be left empty. According to a more recent Tibetan tradition, one-half the volume of the stomach should be filled with solid food, one-fourth with fluid, and one-fourth should remain empty.

In Tibetan medical literature there is a confluence of two major streams of medical knowledge. One stream traces back to *The Four Tantras,* taught by the Buddha himself. These teachings from India were integrated with the indigenous medical knowledge that Tibetans acquired more than two thousand years ago, well before Buddhism was introduced into Tibet. In terms of the proportions of food and drink, the former tradition traces back to the original Indian texts, namely *The Four Tantras,* and I personally feel this classic tradition is superior, for a large intake of fluids helps the blood.

One-fourth of the stomach should remain empty, for this enhances the circulation of the winds. If one has a generally strong digestive warmth, and if one is young and is engaging in much hard physical work, one may eat greater quantities of heavy food. Moreover, after one has eaten, one may drink to one's heart's content, which is to say, until one's thirst is quenched. Drinking large quantities of liquids helps the first stage of the digestive process involving the decomposing phlegm, it enhances the strength of the body, and helps prevent various types of upper chest and throat disorders, such as the common cold. By drinking too little, the decomposing phlegm does not function properly. This produces excessive sputum, which leads to problems in the throat and respiratory disorders.

After eating meat, a person with poor digestive warmth should drink some beer, especially barley beer, for it has a warming quality that aids the digestive process. Moreover, after eating food that is difficult to digest, those with poor digestive warmth should drink hot, boiled water, for this, too, aids the digestive warmth. If one is thin and wants to put on some weight, one should drink beer after a meal; if one is obese and wants to lose weight, after a meal one should drink hot boiled water or herbal tea with honey (not maple syrup).

Generally speaking, during a meal, if one eats and drinks intermittently and in moderation, this helps maintain one's weight right where it is; drinking fluids after a meal results in weight gain; and if one completely slakes one's thirst before a meal, and then drinks nothing more for at least an hour after the meal, one will lose weight. The above general advice about drinking during, before, and after a meal originates from the classical Indian treatises, whereas the advice about drinking honey mixed with hot water stems from the ancient, indigenous tradition of Tibet. If one is serious about losing weight, one should drink hot water (or herbal tea) with honey before the meal, and then drink nothing for at least one hour afterwards. This advice combining both those lineages is doubly effective for losing weight.

Eating healthy foods in moderation helps prevent imbalances of the three humors, enhances the digestive warmth, gives a sense of a lightness of the body, good appetite, clear sensory faculties, and physical strength, and it aids the processes of defecation and urination. This is because it helps the descending wind function properly. For these reasons, one should learn the appropriate amounts of food and drink to ingest and put that knowledge into practice.

Questions and Responses

QUESTION: What do you think of the prospects for integrating modern Western and traditional Tibetan medicine? Specifically, how might we in the West benefit from Tibetan medicine, and how might Tibetans benefit from modern Western medicine?

REPONSE (with a broad smile): This planet on which we live is composed of the five elements, which are the same, whether you are living in Tibet or the United States. We are essentially one people; the color of our skin is of marginal significance. We are one human race on one planet. There will certainly be an integration of these two systems in the West, and people well trained in each one will certainly have much to learn from the others. This is happening already in Asia. I have witnessed it myself in India. When Tibetans fall ill, they may first go to a Western-trained medical doctor to receive initial, fast-acting treatment; but for long-term treatment, they still tend to take Tibetan herbal medication, which works more gradually. There are, of course, some Tibetans who invariably choose only one system or the other, but the integration of these two medical systems is already taking place in practice. There is no question in my mind that people well trained in each of these systems have much to learn from each other. We are, after all, one human race living together on the same planet.

Tibetan medicine can be especially effective in treating various types of wind disorders, including a wide range of disorders of the nervous system. The existence of these winds, or vital energies, is not even acknowledged in modern medicine, so it tends to be weak in this area. For example, from a Tibetan perspective, multiple sclerosis and Parkinson's disease are both wind disorders, for which Western medication is not particularly effective, whereas Tibetan medication can be very helpful. Tibetan medicine has also proven effective for many bile disorders, including hepatitis, which can be completely cured. On the other hand, in the case of serious infections and trauma, as in the case of automobile accidents, Western medicine is the best system on the planet. In such cases, one should take Western medical treatment first, and if some problem lingers after such treatment, one may take Tibetan medicine, which works slowly but may heal the problem from the source.

QUESTION: Americans like ice-cold drinks. Is this healthy, or should drinks be at room temperature or warmer?

RESPONSE: This depends on where you live. If you live in a cold climate, like the Rocky Mountain states or New England, it is unhealthy to drink cold drinks with one's meal. On the other hand, if you live in a warm climate, like California or Florida, you may have cold drinks with your meal, but only in accordance with your digestive warmth. If you drink cold liquids slowly together with your solid food, this will not lead to weight gain or to weight loss.

QUESTION: Are Tibetan doctors, including yourself, aware of detrimental side-effects on the endocrine system and so forth due to the various types of pesticides, herbicides, and other contaminants in our food, water, and air; and do you have ways of counteracting these harmful effects?

RESPONSE: As I commented previously, our situation in the modern era, with the many contaminants introduced into the environment, was prophesied many centuries ago by the Buddha in the medical *tantras*. This prophesy is about an era in which many "ideological extremists" would hold false views, such as materialism, and these people would introduce artificial contaminants into the environment, which would give rise to unprecedented illnesses. There were no cases of these diseases during the time of the Buddha. Nowadays, such artificial contaminants and pollutants are used not only in the West but throughout the world. Traditional Tibetans still avoid the use of herbicides and pesticides on their crops, but if they have to buy food that has been contaminated with them, they wash them and try to wait a week or two before consuming them in the hope that some of the contaminants will evaporate. The twentieth century is the era prophesied as a time when such contaminants will lead to various microbial and infectious diseases; and the classic Indian Buddhist medical treatises explain the origins, nature, and ways of treating those diseases. The first classification of them includes eighteen illnesses, but those are subdivided into more than forty diseases.

When I was a child in Tibet, occasionally some Western foods, such as candy, would be brought to my village, but the Tibetan elders would encourage us children not to eat this wrapped and processed food, cautioning us that it was probably contaminated. Learned Tibetans have known for centuries that there would come a time when such contaminants would be introduced into foods, so they have been wary. Nowadays, though, as the decades have gone by, many Tibetans have grown accustomed to processed Western food and they enjoy it.

When I was about nineteen and had completed my formal medical training at the Tibetan Medical Institute in Lhasa, from about nine to ten o'clock every morning I would go to the British-operated clinic called Dekyi Ling. This adjoined the British Trade Mission, led by Hugh Richardson and inhabited by other Englishmen as well. I would go to their clinic to learn some Western medical procedures, including first aid, injections, and the use of antibiotics. When I was there, they would offer visitors candy. I would accept it and show it to the older Tibetans, telling them, "This is English food, and if you eat it, you will get English diseases." Other Tibetans didn't like it and didn't want to touch it. When India won independence from Britain in 1947, this trade mission was turned over to the Indian government. Then a number of Indians, some of them from Sikkim, moved in, and they spoke a dialect of Tibetan so we could converse quite easily. They, too, brought with them processed foods such as candy and tinned meat. As I spent time with them, I got into the habit of eating their food, which I came to enjoy, but when I showed it to the older Tibetans, they were suspicious and didn't want to touch it. They thought the meat might be dog meat or even human meat, for they thought that Westerners might be cannibals. Older Tibetans were generally very conservative about Western foods and would not eat, or even have in their homes, beef, poultry, or pork. The only meat they would eat was mutton and yak meat. Since the Chinese Communist invasion of Tibet, the Chinese have brought their own dietary customs. The Tibetans under Chinese rule have adapted to them, and many will now eat poultry, pork, beef and anything else the Chinese eat.

QUESTION: You spoke of two types of enemas, a mild laxative and a strong purgative. Among the enemas presently available in the West, are there any that you know of that might be helpful for wind disorders? Or are there herbs that we in the West could put to use right now to help people with wind disorders?

RESPONSE: Yes. Both wild and cultivated ginger, for example, can be very useful in this regard. The three types of the mild Tibetan laxatives have many ingredients, but I don't think it would be wise for people to ingest these without knowing the proper proportions and ways of compounding them. The strong Tibetan purgative is easy to prepare, but the mild laxatives have more ingredients and are more difficult to make.

QUESTION: Do medications for wind disorders, which generally seem to have some relation to the nervous system, have a more direct effect on the brain than medications for phlegm and bile disorders?

RESPONSE: Yes, this is generally true. The reason is that the pervading wind is located in the head, and it contributes to all types of voluntary motions of the limbs and so on. Any disorder of the pervading wind affects the entire body, even though it is located in the head, so medication to alleviate disorders of the pervading wind would of course influence the brain. Generally, the health and functioning of the body as a whole are especially related to the winds and their circulation. Blood circulates through the body because of the wind humor. Just as an engine is needed to power a hydraulic pump, so does the wind humor power the heart to pump blood. The heart by itself is just a muscle, but it is the wind humor that enables it to perform its function of circulating the blood, and wind moves other fluids throughout the body as well.

Among the five types of winds, the life-sustaining wind is located in the heart; but medication for disorders of this type of wind affects not only the heart but the brain as well. Generally speaking, if the wind humor is functioning properly, the body as a whole will be in good health, and if the winds are imbalanced, this impairs one's general state of health. The winds are also especially closely related to the functioning of the senses, so this also relates them to the brain. The classical Tibetan medical texts state that the five hundred types of channels (including veins, arteries, and nerves) are closely related to the five physical senses as well as mental functions such as alertness and memory; and all those channels are directly related to the brain.

QUESTION: Does the Tibetan medical tradition include the practices of acupressure, acupuncture, shiatsu, or moxibustion on the various nodal points?

RESPONSE (with laughter): There are five categories of Tibetan medicine pertaining to those modes of treatment. First of all, three types of moxibustion are widely practiced in the Tibetan tradition. Long ago, a system of acupuncture originated in Tibet and from there it was brought to Mongolia and on to China. The Chinese extended and elaborated this method of treatment, but it actually originated in Tibet. Tibetan medicine also includes blood-letting and a general category of massage using various types of ointments for specific ailments. Hot and cold poultices, hot mineral baths, and immersion in hot springs are also practiced. If one has a wind disorder, massages using medicinal ointments can be especially helpful. If one has a bile disorder, one should relax and avoid rigorous hard work. If one has a phlegm disorder, various types of *yoga* exercises may be helpful.

QUESTION: First, what is your opinion about radiation therapy; and second, what do you think of the effect of radiation introduced into the environment? Many Native Americans believe that uranium should stay in the earth, where its presence is thought to help produce rain. What is your position?

RESPONSE: Radiation therapy is part of the Western medical tradition, and when oncologists feel it is necessary to use it to treat cancer, they will do so, regardless of what I think. From my own experience, however, I believe it would be better if radiation were not used in the initial phases of treatment of breast cancer, for example, but only in the final phases of treatment. Some years ago, I knew a woman with breast cancer in the left breast who had a lumpectomy. Afterwards a large lesion and swelling appeared on the right side of her chest. Her doctors told her there was no way to treat this and that she had only five months to live. She then came to me for treatment, and I first gave her medication for one month. During that time, the swelling became significantly smaller and the lesion was healing. I then advised her to return to France, where she lived, and request radiation treatment from her physician. She did so, and following the radiation therapy, the lesion healed. Now, a year later, she is still alive. I think that was one instance in which radiation was helpful.

Radiation treatment destroys bodily tissue, and radiation introduced into the environment is likewise potentially lethal. But radiation, like just about everything else in nature, can be beneficial or harmful, depending on how it's used. The traditional Tibetan view accords with the belief of the native Americans, who are originally of Tibetan stock, concerning the relationship between uranium in the ground and rain. The Bön tradition, the indigenous religion of Tibet prior to the introduction of Buddhism in Tibet, asserts that glowing, or radiating, minerals are conducive to rain. So they should be left in the ground, and if they are unearthed, they should be covered over again with soil. It is believed that if one makes use of such minerals, this leads to harmful results. This appears to accord with the Native American belief. However, with the Chinese occupation of Tibet, the Chinese are mining uranium as fast as they can and using it for energy and weapons.

Before the Chinese invasion, when there were still British emissaries in Tibet, the British did some prospecting in Tibet and found uranium deposits. They also found gold deposits in my home region in southern Tibet, which they marked. They then petitioned the Tibetan government to mine these minerals, and in return they offered to build a bridge across the Tsangpo River, which Tibetans would cross in small coracles. They assured the Tibetans that such a bridge would be good for everybody. But the Tibetans refused, saying they didn't want the mining or the bridge. When the Chinese came, they continued the prospecting begun by the British, and now they are mining those uranium and gold deposits.

CONCLUDING COMMENT: I deeply appreciate the interest so many Westerners have shown in Tibetan medicine. I would especially encourage young Westerners interested in this medical system to study the Tibetan language. If you can both speak and read Tibetan, you can learn from Tibetan medical practitioners and other scholars of the Tibetan tradition, and you can have access to the vast body of Tibetan literature on medicine and other topics. These texts are available not only in Asia but in many university libraries in the United States. The texts are available; the only thing missing is Westerners able to read them! So I encourage all of you who are sincerely interested in this medical tradition to learn the language so you can study it well. From my heart I thank you for your interest in our medical heritage!

English-Tibetan-Sanskrit Medical Glossary

English	Tibetan	Sanskrit
accomplishing bile	mkhris pa sgrub byed	sādhaka-pitta
acne	khye ma	
aconite poisoning	btsan dug	vatsanābha-viṣa
afflicted elements	gnod bya'i khams	dūṣya-dhātu
afflictions	nyes pa	doṣa
afflictive elements	gnod byed kyi khams	duṣṭikāra-dhātu
agitated heat disorder	'khrugs tshad	śrana-jvara
air poisoning	rdzi dug	vāyu-duṣṭi
ambrosial pill	bdud rtsi ril bu	
amnesia	brjed byed	apasmāra
anemia	skya rbab	pāṇḍu-roga
anuria	gcin 'gags	mūtrāghāta
aphrodisiac	ro tsa	
ascending wind	rlung gyen rgyu	udāna-vāyu
ascites	dmu chu	jalodara
asthma	dbugs mi bde	śvāsa-roga
bile	mkhris pa	pitta
blister	shu ba	visphoṭaka
blood and ovum	khrag	rakta
bodily constituent	lus zungs	dhātu
bone-spur	rus lhag	
brain	klad pa	mastuluṅga

brown phlegm	bad kan smug po	
bubbly tumor of the uterus	mngal skran chu bur can	
cartilage	khrum rus	
cerumen	rna sbabs	
cervical lymphadenitis (?)	'bras	apacī
chebulic myrobalan (*Terminalia chebula*)	a ru ra rnam rgyal	haritaki
cholera	tshad 'khru	jvara-atisāra
colic pain	glan thabs	śūla-roga
color-transforming bile	mkhris pa mdangs sgyur	rañjaka-pitta
complexion-clearing bile	mkhris pa mdog gsal	bhrājaka-pitta
common cold	cham pa	pratiśyāya
connective phlegm	bad kan 'byor byed	śleṣaka-kapha
constipation	rtug 'gags	koṣṭhabaddha
costus root (*Saussurea lappa: Costus speciosus*)	ru rta	
cyst; lymph node; lipoma; nodule mass	rmen bu	granthi
cystoid tumor	rmen skran	
dangling tumor of the channels	rtsa skran ling ba	
dark channel	rtsa nag	śirā śotha
dark residual tumor	skran ro nag po	
decomposing phlegm	bad kan myag byed	kledaka-kapha
dependent edema	'or	śotha
depletion	zad pa	
descending wind	rlung thur sel	apāna-vāyu
detrimental side-effect	log pa	
developing heat disorder	rgyas tshad	
diarrhea	khru	atisāra
diaphragm	mchin dri	
digestive bile	mkhris pa 'ju byed	pācaka-pitta
digestive warmth	me drod	agni
disease due to airborn poison	rlung gi rdzi dug	
disease due to the sun's radiation	nyi zer gyi dug	

dysphagia, anorexia	yid ga 'chus pa	arocaka
dysuria	gcin snyi	mūtra-kṛcchra
eaglewood or aloewood (*Aquilaria agallocha*)	a ga ru	agaru
eczema or ichthyosis	glang shu	vicarcikā
elephantiasis	rkang 'bam	ślīpada
empty heat disorder	stongs tshad	
erysipelas	me dbal	visarpa
experiencing phlegm	bad kan myong byed	bodhaka-kapha
extrasensory perception	mngon shes	abhijñā
extreme thirst	skom dad	tṛṣṇā-roga
eye excretion	mig skyag	
fast-acting purgative enema	ni ru ha	nirūha
fire-accompanying wind	rlung me mnyam	samāna-vāyu
firm blood tumor	khrag skran hrem po	
food poisoning	mi 'phrod pa'i dug	asātmya-āhāra-viṣa
four immeasurables	tshad med bzhi	catvāryapramāṇi
frozen disorder; frozen tumor	hreng po	
goiter	lba ba	gala-gaṇḍa
gout	dreg nad	vāta-rakta
granulated spheres as holy relics	ring bsrel	
groin	sne khud	
heart wind	snying rlung	
hemorrhoid	gzhang 'brum	arśas
hepatomegali	'chin babs	
hiccups	skyigs bu	hikkā-roga
hidden heat disorder	gab tshad	
hip joint	dpyi mig	
hollow organs	snod	suṣirāśaya
hot swelling; the microorganism responsible for this disease	lhog pa	visphoṭaka
humor	nad	doṣa
humors	nyes pa	doṣa
Indian bedellium tree (*Commiphora mukul*)	gu gul	

indestructible *bindu*	mi shigs pa'i thig le	
indigestion	ma zhu	agnimāndya
infectious disease	rims nad	saṇkrāmaka-jvara
insanity	smyo byed	unmāda
insect poisoning	srin bu dug	vṛścika-viṣa
insensitive tumor of the flesh	sha skran bem po	
internal lesion	sur ya	āmāśaya-vraṇa
invasion	zhugs pa	
kama, canonical teachings of the Buddha	bka' ma	
leprosy	mdze	kuṣṭha
leucoderma	sha bkra	
life-force channel	srog rtsa	prāṇa-nāḍi
life-force	srog	
life-sustaining wind	rlung srog 'dzin	prāṇa-vāyu
luster	mdangs	
lymph; serous fluid	chu ser	lasīkā
manufactured poison	sbyar dug	kṛtrima-viṣa
meat poisoning	sha dug	māṃsa-viṣa
microbial disease	gnyan	kṛcchra
microbial and infectious diseases	gnyan rims	
mild laxative	'jam rtsi	anuvāsana basti
mixed heat disorder	rnyog tshad	
mole	dme ba	
moment	thang	kalā?
mustard seed	yungs kar	
nutriment (plasma & chyle?)	dangs ma	rasa
oily film (on surface of urine)	spris ma	
oral lineage	gang zag snyan rgyud	
organism	srin	
ovum tumor	sa bon skran	
perineal fistula	mtshan bar rdol ba	bhagandara
pervading wind	rlung khyab byed	vyāna-vāyu
phase	yud tsam	muhūrtta

phlegm	bad kan	kapha
poisoning from snakebite	sbrul gyi dug	sarpa-viṣa
potency	nus pa	virya
precious pill	rin chen ril bu	
pregnancy mask and other skin disorders	ngo khabs	mukha-dūṣikā
protection from infection	rims srung	
pustule	thor pa	
quality	yon tan	guṇa
rabies	khyi dug	alarka-viṣa
racing blood	khrag tshabs	
rectum	gnye ma	
red element	khams dmar po	
regenerative substance (sperm & uterine blood, or ovum)	khu ba	śukra
residue	snyigs ma	
rheumatoid arthritis	grum bu	sandhi-vāta
ringworm (?)	za kong	dadru
satisfying phlegm	bad kan tshim byed	tarpaka-kapha
scabies (?)	g.yan pa	kaṇḍū
sclera	mig sprin	
sebum	dreg pa	
sequentially compounded disorder	bla gnyan	
serious chronic disease	gcong chen ati-jirṇa	rāja yakṣmā
seven wondrous pulses	ngo mtshar rtsa bdun	
sexually-transmitted diseases	reg pa'i dug	kacchu
shooting pains in the small intestines	rgyu zer	āntra-śūla or pravāhikā
sight-giving bile	mkhris pa mthong byed	ālocaka-pitta
simultaneous, compound disorder	'doms pa	
six perfections	pha rol tu phyin pa drug	ṣaṭ-pāramitā
smallpox	'brum bu	masūrikā
solid organs	don	saṃhatāśaya

spinal cord	rgyungs pa	
splendor	gzi brjid	
spreading heat disorder	'grams tshad	kṣata-kṣaya
supportive phlegm	bad kan rten byed	avalambaka-kapha
suspended sediment (in urine)	ku ya	
sweet flag (*Acorus calamus*)	shu dag	
tantric adept	sngags pa	mantrin
terma; "treasure teaching"	gter ma	
thoraco-lumbar fascia	bshul sha	
tonic (medicinal butter)	sman mar	
tumor	skran	gulma
upper chest, neck, and head	nam tshong	
urticaria	bas ldags	kotha
vapor poisoning	rlang dug	vāṣpa-viṣa
vesicle of regenerative substances = seminal vesicle & ovaries	bsam bse'u	śukrāśaya ḍimbāśaya
vital essence	bcud	rasa
vital essence medicine	bcud len	
vitality	tshe	āyus
vomiting	skyug	vamana
warts	mdzer pa	
waste product	dri ma	mala
white channel	rtsa dkar	śveta-nāḍi
white element	khams dkar po	
wild turkey	bya ngar	
wind	rlung	vāyu, vāta
womb; ovaries, uterus, and breasts	mngal	
xiphoid	lhan	
zaku blood tumor	khrag skran za khu	
zee stone	gzi rdo	

Tibetan-English-Sanskrit Medical Glossary

English	Tibetan	Sanskrit
ku ya	suspended sediment (in urine)	
khye ma	acne	
klad pa	brain	mastuluṅga
bka' ma	kama, canonical teachings of the Buddha	
rkang 'bam	elephantiasis	ślīpada
skom dad	extreme thirst	tṛṣṇā-roga
skya rbab	anemia	pāṇḍu-roga
skyigs bu	hiccups	hikkā-roga
skyug	vomiting	vamana
skran	tumor	gulma
skran ro nag po	dark residual tumor	
khams dkar po	white element	
khams dmar po	red element	
khu ba	regenerative substance (sperm & uterine blood or ovum)	śukra
khyi dug	rabies	alarka-viṣa
khrag	uterine blood, or ovum	rakta
khrag skran hrem po	firm blood tumor	
khrag tshabs	racing blood	

khrag skran za khu	*zaku* blood tumor	
khru	diarrhea	atisāra
khrum rus	cartilage	
mkhris pa	bile	pitta
mkhris pa sgrub byed	accomplishing bile	sādhaka-pitta
mkhris pa 'ju byed	digestive bile	pācaka-pitta
mkhris pa mthong byed	sight-giving bile	ālocaka-pitta
mkhris pa mdangs sgyur	color-transforming bile	rañjaka-pitta
mkhris pa mdog gsal	complexion-clearing bile	bhrājaka-pitta
'khrugs tshad	agitated heat disorder	śrana-jvara
gang zag snyan rgyud	oral lineage	
gab tshad	hidden heat disorder	
gu gul	Indian bedellium tree (*Commiphora mukul*)	
grum bu	rheumatoid arthritis	sandhi-vāta
glang shu	eczema or ichthyosis	vicarcikā
glan thabs	colic pain	śūla-roga
'grams tshad	spreading heat disorder	kṣata-kṣaya
rgyas tshad	developing heat disorder	
rgyu zer	shooting pains in the small intestine	āntra-śūla or pravāhikā
rgyungs pa	spinal cord	
ngo khabs	pregnancy mask and other skin disorders	mukha-dūṣikā
ngo mtshar rtsa bdun	seven wondrous pulses	
mngal	womb; may also refer to the ovaries, uterus, and breasts	
mngal skran chu bur can	bubbly tumor of the uterus	
mngon shes	extrasensory perception	abhijñā
sngags pa	tantric adept	mantrin
gcin 'gags	anuria	mūtrāghāta
gcin snyi	dysuria	mūtra-kṛcchra
cong chen	serious chronic disease	rāja yakṣmā ati-jirṇa
bcud	vital essence	rasa
bcud len	vital essence medicine	
cham pa	common cold	pratiśyāya

chu ser	lymph; serous fluid	lasīkā
mchin dri	diaphragm	
'chin babs	hepatomegali	
'jam rtsi	mild laxative	anuvāsana basti
brjed byed	amnesia	apasmāra
nyi zer gyi dug	disease due to the sun's radiation	aṃśu-viṣa
nyes pa	afflictions, humors	doṣa
gnyan	microbial disease	kṛcchra
gnyan rims	microbial and infectious diseases	
gnye ma	rectum	
rnyog tshad	mixed heat disorder	
snyigs ma	residue	
snying rlung	heart wind	
gter ma	terma; "treasure teaching"	
rtug 'gags	constipation	koṣṭhabaddha
stongs tshad	empty heat disorder	
thang	moment	kalā?
thor pa	pustule	
dangs ma	nutriment (plasma & chyle?)	rasa
don	solid organs	saṃhatāśaya
dvangs ma	nutriment	rasa
dri ma	waste product	mala
dreg nad	gout	vāta-rakta
dreg pa	sebum	
bdud rtsi ril bu	ambrosial pill	
mdangs	luster	
'doms pa	simultaneous, compound disorder	
nad	humor	doṣa
nam tshong	upper chest, neck, and head	
ni ru ha	a fast-acting purgative enema	nirūha
nus pa	potency	virya
gnod bya'i khams	afflicted elements	dūṣya-dhātu

gnod byed kyi khams	afflictive elements	duṣṭikāra-dhātu
rna sbabs	cerumen	
sne khud	groin	
snod	hollow organs	suṣirāśaya
dpyi mig	hip joint	
spris ma	oily film (on surface of urine)	
pha rol tu phyin pa drug	six perfections	saṭ-pāramitā
bad kan	phlegm	kapha
bad kan rten byed	supportive phlegm	avalambaka-kapha
bad kan 'byor byed	connective phlegm	śleṣaka-kapha
bad kan myag byed	decomposing phlegm	kledaka-kapha
bad kan myong byed	experiencing phlegm	bodhaka-kapha
bad kan smug po	brown phlegm	
bad kan tshim byed	satisfying phlegm	tarpaka-kapha
bas ldags	urticaria	kotha
bya ngar	wild turkey	
bla gnyan	sequentially compounded disorder	
dbugs mi bde	asthma	śvāsa-roga
'bras	cervical lymphadenitis (?)	apacī
'brum bu	smallpox	masūrikā
lba ba	goiter	gala-gaṇḍa
sbyar dug	manufactured poison	kṛtrima-viṣa
sbrul gyi dug	poisoning from snake-bite	sarpa-viṣa
ma zhu	indigestion	agnimāndya
mi 'phrod pa'i dug	food poisoning	asātmya-āhāra-viṣa
mi shigs pa'i thig le	indestructible *bindu*	
mig skyag	eye excretion	
mig sprin	sclera	
me drod	digestive warmth	agni
me dbal	erysipelas	visarpa
dmu chu	ascites	jalodara
dme ba	mole	
rmen skran	cystoid tumor	
rmen bu	cyst, subcutaneous nodule, lipoma	granthi
sman mar	tonic (medicinal butter)	

rmen bu	cyst; lymph node; lipoma; nodule mass	
smyo byed	insanity	unmāda
btsan dug	aconite poisoning	vatsanābha-viṣa
rtsa skran ling ba	dangling tumor of the channels	
rtsa dkar	white channel	śveta-nāḍi
rtsa nag	dark channel	śirā śotha
tshe	vitality	āyus
tshad 'khru	cholera	jvara-atisāra
tshad med bzhi	four immeasurables	catvāryapramāṇi
mtshan bar rdol ba	perineal fistula	bhagandara
mdze	leprosy	kuṣṭha
mdzer pa	warts	
rdzi dug	air poisoning	vāyu-duṣṭi
zhugs pa	invasion	
gzhang 'brum	hemorrhoid	arśas
za kong	ring-worm (?)	dadru
zad pa	depletion	
gzi brjid	splendor	
gzi rdo	*zee* stone	
'or	dependent edema	śotha
yid ga 'chus pa	dysphagia, anorexia	arocaka
yud tsam	phase	muhūrtta
yungs kar	mustard seed	
yon tan	quality	guṇa
g.yan pa	scabies (?)	kaṇḍū
ring bsrel	granulated spheres as holy relics	
rin chen ril bu	precious pill	
rims nad	infectious disease	saṇkrāmaka-jvara
rims srung	protection from infection	
ru rta	costus root (*Saussurea lappa; Costus speciosus*)	
rus lhag	bone-spur	
reg pa'i dug	sexually-transmitted diseases, literally "diseases from contact"	kacchu

ro tsa	aphrodisiac	
rlang dug	vapor poisoning	vāṣpa-viṣa
rlung	wind	vāyu, vāta
rlung khyab byed	pervading wind	vyāna-vāyu
rlung gi rdzi dug	disease due to airborn poison	
rlung gyen rgyu	ascending wind	udāna-vāyu
rlung thur sel	descending wind	apāna-vāyu
rlung me mnyam	fire-accompanying wind	samāna-vāyu
rlung srog 'dzin	life-sustaining wind	prāṇa-vāyu
lus zungs	bodily constituent	dhātu
log pa	detrimental side-effect	
sha bkra	leucoderma	
sha skran bem po	insensitive tumor of the flesh	
sha dug	meat poisoning	māṃsa-viṣa
shu dag	sweet flag (*Acorus calamus*)	
shu ba	blister	visphoṭaka
bshul sha	thoraco-lumbar fascia	
sa bon skran	ovum tumor	
sur ya	internal lesion	āmāśaya-vraṇa
srin	organism	
srin bu dug	insect poisoning	vṛścika-viṣa
srog	life-force	prāṇa
srog rtsa	life-force channel	
bsam bse'u	vesicle of regenerative substances = seminal vesicle & ovaries	śukrāśaya ḍimbāśaya
hreng po	frozen disorder; frozen tumor	
lhan	xiphoid	
lhog pa	hot swelling; the micro-organism responsible for this disease	visphoṭaka
a ga ru	eaglewood or aloewood (*Aquilaria agallocha*)	agaru
a ru ra rnam rgyal	chebulic myrobalan (*Terminalia chebula*)	haritaki

Glossary of Names

Amdo	A mdo
Bihla Gadzey	Bi lha dga' mdzes
Biji Gadjé	Bi byi dga' byed
Bodhgaya	rDo rje gdan
Bön	Bon
Choka Chejor	Co ka bcad byor
Chokrong Lü Gyaltsen	lCog rong klu'i rgyal mtshan
Darmo Lobzang Chödrak	Dar mo blo bzang chos grags
Degé	bDe dge
Dekyi Ling	bDe skyid gling
Drapa Ngönshey	Grwa pa mngon shes
Drejey Vajra	'Dre rje vajra
Dunggi Thorchok	gDung gi mthor cog
Jamyang Shäpa	'Jam dbyangs bshad pa
Jangpa	Byang pa
Jigmé Wangpo	'Jigs med dbang po
Kachupa	bKa' bcu pa
kama	bka' ma
Khyenrab Norbu	mKhyen rab nor bu
Khyenrab Ösel	mKhyen rab 'od gsal
Khyungpo	Khyung po
Kumbum	sKu 'bum
Lodrö Shenyen	bLo gros bshes gnyen

Manasija, "Mind-born"	Yid las skyes
Mangsong Mangtsen	Mang srong mang btsan
Me Agtsom	Mes ag tshom
Ngok Chöku Dorje	rNgog chos sku rdo rje
Paṇḍit Candradeva	Mkhas pa Mi dbang
Potramo	Po spra mo
Regent Sangye Gyatso	sDe srid sangs rgyas rgya mtsho
Rapjampa	Rab 'byams pa
Rinchen Zangpo	Rin chen bzang po
Sangye Gyatso	Sangs rgyas rgya mtsho
Satyakathāsiddhi, "The Adept Whose Words of Truth Come True"	Drang srong bden tshig sgrub pa
Sönam Wangden	bSod nams dbang ldan
Songtsen Gampo	Srong btsan sgam po
Sungrab Ling	gSung rab gling
Sudarśana, "Lovely to Behold"	lTa na sdug
Tashi Kyil	bKra shis dkyil
Thönmi Sambhoṭa	Thon mi Sambhoṭa
Thothori Nyentsen	Tho tho ri gnyan brtsan
Trisong Detsen	Khri srong lde btsan
Vaidyarāja, "Sovereign Healer"	sMan pa'i rgyal po
Vidyājñāna, "Primordial Wisdom of Awareness"	Rig pa'i ye shes
Yeshi Dhonden	Ye shes don ldan
Yikyi Rölcha	Yid kyi rol cha
Yumbu Lagang	Yum bu bla sgang
Yuthok Yönten Gönpo	gYu thog yon tan mgon po
Zurpa	Zur pa

Glossary of Texts

The Ancestral Oral Tradition
Mes po'i zhal lung

Blue Vaiḍūrya
Bai ḍūr ya sngon po

The Explanatory Tantra
bShad rgyud
Ākhyāta-tantra

The Final Tantra
Phyi ma'i rgyud
Uttara-tantra

The Four Tantras
rGyud bzhi
Catuḥ-tantra

The Hundred Works of Darma
Dar ma bka' rgya ma

Kālacakra-tantra
Dus kyi 'khor lo'i rgyud

The Oral Instruction Tantra
Man ngag rgyud
Upadeśa-tantra

The Root Tantra
rTsa rgyud
Mūla-tantra

The Stainless Light
Dri med 'od
Vimalaprabhā

Supplement to The Oral Instruction Tantra
Man ngag lhan thabs

Bibliography

Asaṅga & Tsong-Kha-Pa. (1986) Asanga's Chapter on Ethics with the Commentary of Tsong-Kha-Pa, *The Basic Path to Awakening*, The Complete Bodhisattva. trans. Mark Tatz. Lewiston: Edwin Mellen Press. Studies in Asian Thought and Religion, Vol. 4.

Blo bzang hstan 'dzin. *Bod kyi gso rig slob deb*. Dharamsala: Bod gzhung sman rtsis khang gso rig mtho slob sde tshan.

Clark, Barry, trans. (1995) *The Quintessence Tantras of Tibetan Medicine*. Ithaca: Snow Lion.

Dash, Vaidya Bhagwan. (1994) *Encyclopedia of Tibetan Medicine*. Delhi: Sri Satguru Publications.

mGon po dbang rgyal. (1986) *Chos kyi rnam grangs*. Chengdu: Sichuan People's Press.

Lamrimpa, Gen. (1995) *Calming the Mind: Tibetan Buddhist Teachings on Cultivating Meditative Quiescence*, trans. B. Alan Wallace. Ithaca: Snow Lion.

Lamrimpa, Gen. (1999) *Realizing Emptiness: The Madhyamaka Cultivation of Insight*, trans. B. Alan Wallace, ed. Ellen Posman. Ithaca: Snow Lion.

Lamrimpa, Gen. (1999) *Transcending Time: An Explanation of the Kālacakra Six-Session Guruyoga*, trans. B. Alan Wallace, ed. Pauly Fitze. Boston: Wisdom.

Padmasambhava. (1998) *Natural Liberation: Padmasambhava's Teachings on the Six Bardos*, comm. by Gyatrul Rinpoche; trans. by B. Alan Wallace. Boston: Wisdom.

Śāntideva. (1997) *A Guide to the Bodhisattva Way of Life*. trans. Vesna A. Wallace & B. Alan Wallace. Ithaca: Snow Lion.

Sogyal Rinpoche. (1992) *The Tibetan Book of Living and Dying*. San Francisco: Harper SanFrancisco.

Tse tan zhab drung, Dung dkar blo bzang phrin las, & dMu dge bsam gtan. (1984) *Bod rgya tshig mdzod chen mo*, Mi rigs dpe skrun khang (People's Publishing House), 3 vols.

Wallace, B. Alan. (1998) *The Bridge of Quiescence: Experiencing Tibetan Buddhist Meditation.* Chicago: Open Court.

Wallace, B. Alan. (1999) *Boundless Heart: The Four Immeasurables.* Ithaca: Snow Lion.

Dr. Yeshi Donden. (1986) *Health Through Balance*, ed. & trans. by Jeffrey Hopkins. Ithaca: Snow Lion.

Index